AfriKan Yoga

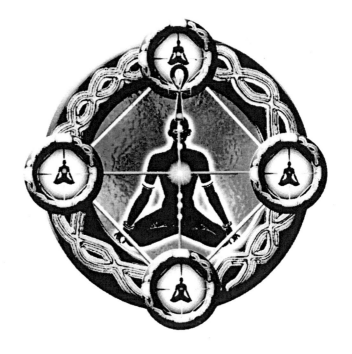

The Re-Emergence of
TAMARE SMAI TAUI

A Practical Guide to Wellbeing through Smai
Posture, Breath and Meditation

AfriKan Yoga

A Practical Guide to Wellbeing through Smai Posture, Breath and Meditation

Published in 2008 by TamaRe House Publishers Ltd
www.tamarehouse.com
info@tamarehouse.com

Printed and Bound by Lightning Source, Milton Keynes, UK

Authored by Pablo M. Imani

ISBN: 978-1-906169-40-4

Contents

AfriKan Yoga

Dedication

To my deities in the flesh, the children who blessed me: Kha'mara, (Black Sun) Nefertem (Beautiful Completion) and Amenta (Keeper of The Secrets). You are so good for me; you have expanded me and continue to do so, may you find your true paths.

To the Smai students and Afrikan Yogis everywhere, come home.

To those who are awakening; welcome, let's work together.

Acknowledgements

Thanks to NETER; I am nothing but a vessel of your divine will.

The Neteru Ancestors, ancient and modern; I thank you each and everyday with all my being. You strengthen my, body, soul and spirit. You reside in my being because when I look within, all I see is your boundless blackness. When I look without all I see is your supreme manifestations. Thank you truly for the personification of Smai Afrikan Yoga, as a science of reconnecting, and the personification of this book.

The Supreme GrandMaster Teacher AmunNubi RuakhPtah...
Thank you for accepting me as a student in the Ancient Mystic Order of Melchizedek and the Ancient Egiptian Order. Since the day we met your enthusiasm and humility has always struck a resounding chord for me. Thank you for raising me from the mentally dead and inspiring me with your words, deeds and tireless work. You wrote over 360 books and planted seeds in thousands, which signifies Tehuti incarnate. You showed me that it is possible to incarnate our great blood seed ancestors, Pa Neters, here and now. You made terms like 'Right Knowledge' common amongst Africans in the Diaspora. You are the A'aferti (Pharaoh) in this day and time. You taught me not to be afraid to be different; to accept my opposing natures and unify them (Smai Tawi). Your spirit cannot be contained for it is here with us around the globe. This work is indeed a testament to your teaching to which I have attempted to disseminate in the way I was guided to do.

Co-teacher, co-healer, Goddess Ife Piankhi, you are a true djed backbone. You are a living Aset, strength wisdom and beauty in the flesh. I have not been an easy person to walk with and I know I am challenging and intense at times. Thank you for your patience, the conversations, meditations, love and supporting me over the years, and of course my obsessions while writing this piece. Thank you mainly for your love and the deepest understanding I have ever known.

Master Teacher, Dr Muata Ashby, who has inspired me with his writings, works and teachings. You made this possible because without your scholarly works this could not be realised. I hope many Afrikan Yogis choose to study your writings and see for themselves the rich heritage of Afrikan Yoga.

Master Teacher, Dr Imhotep Llaila 'O' Afrika, mentor, friend, patron and teacher who sees my shortcomings yet in his wisdom gently encourages me to stay strong fuses me with 'I can'. You are a General for health; a master warrior healer. Your genius is undisputed. What you have taught in the areas of African traditional medicine, art and sciences, holistic diagnosis and remedies is gigantic.

It has been a pleasure and honour to sit at your feet sir, thank you as I have learnt so much from you.

And to the training through the various schools from back streets, to parks, to the community halls, to classrooms and on the 'road' I have received, which at times admittedly I really struggled with.

In particular I acknowledge all my teachers, in the martial sciences Master Toddy of Muy Thai; I don't think he will remember this rather small child so many years ago. I hear you are doing T.V shows in Thailand. Thanks to my Thai Chi teacher Mac, without the practise of Thai Chi I would not have realised the similarities and the differences between Chinese Thai Chi and Hudu/Afrikan Yoga. Thanks to Sean Lee 'Luwt/Narmer' who introduced me to Wing Chung and our exchange of Taoist teachings. Thanks to brothers KMT for Kilindi 'stick fighting' and Cisco for Capoirera Angola. I really enjoyed our stretching and playfully sessions in my backyard and on Streatham common. You were so encouraging in regards to the yoga, thank you. Thanks to Hamza, Lyon, Levi, Asafo, Batekun, Anwar and all my brothers and sisters in 'Kazimba (*Ka Shill Pa Nefer Akir/Spirit of the Young Lion*) Ngoma' family at the Academy of Nubian Cultural Arts.

I acknowledge The Ancient Egyptian Art Ka-*Akiru (Akh-Heru)* propogated by my brother Ab Ankh Rhem Saiyome Scarlett Hudson 'Karuma'. We have grown and entwined together in brotherhood, in practise and insight, I give thanks to our passionate talks and reasonings on matters such as spirituality, relationships, Love, mind and esoteric knowledge from Afrika. I also acknowledge Batekun now Known as Astehmari, Teacher of Dankira Tawagi 'Warrior Dance'; the reasonings through wordsound and Ngoma as always been a great joy. I thank the Maashufa family, in particular Onyeka and Afua for your work in the Afrikan martial sciences, your support in having my classes at the Nub and also your generosity and support of my family in difficult times. I thank all of you and the sciences you teach that resides in my heart. My wish with the deepest respect is to develop our healing arm and for future practitioners to embrace our Ancient African heritage. *Hashima/Nadebu/ Respect.*

Thanks to Lloyd 'Rez' Parker 'Mr Rezmela-nine/Rezonance for your support in so many ways. Thanks also for introducing me to Qi Gong; the spaces we shared were so edifiying. We really experimented with stretching, breath and healing arts to the point that we literally blacked out. I see that as a death which is the eternal; it was a strange but funny experience and one I enjoyed, thank you for the laughter and the many 'reasonings'.

5

Thank you Darren Teroa Rakaua Tishu Tanu for sharing Ashtanga Yoga with me but mainly for being so supportive as a long time friend; we too have seen much changes in each other over the years. It must be close to 2 decades now. You are a 'Solar Brother' of great stature, so continue to release the Neter within.

Thanks to Stefan Cartwright, a Yoga teacher and Sound healer who saw that I was a yogi before I even realised it my self. I watched you practise and share your pranyama with me on the cliffs of Brighton after a night of deejaying in the clubs of Brighton. Thank you for accepting the rebel that I am; thank you for the understanding and thank you for your acknowledgment. I acknowledge my present studies which are a real spiritual and mental safari; that I feel they're will be no end.

I also want to thank Amasade Shepnekhi of Mothership. I wonder if you realised the morning when you saw me stretching, preparing for Kazimba training and said I was practising yoga, the seed you watered.

Thanks to Iva Polka, mother of nephew Osei and niece Yasu, for introducing me to Hatha Yoga around 20 years ago. Those stretches you taught I have carried with me for so long and very much alive in me. Thank you for watering my seed and I am glad to hear you are still teaching in West London.

Many thanks to my family, my parents Muriel and Edward Samuels, for the strengthening this small wayward boy with bitter herbs, my siblings Norma, Joseph, Veronica, Yvonne, Gloria, Charles (a practitioner of tai chi), Hillman 'Daki', (a practitioner of yoga). Also Daki – this book is for you – because you nurtured and shone on the small Rasta and Afrikan pride seed in me as a young boy; thank you. Doriline, my sister who protected and cared for me in my early years; yeah I know I used to get you into trouble with mom and dad numerous times, sorry for that. I am grateful for our experiences because now I know why I am the ninth child.

I aknowledge my extended family, there are so many of you to mention, cousins, nephews, nieces, great, and great great, in America, Canada, Jamaica, Barbados, Cuba and Panama. To the family I hope to find in Morocco and Mali. One day I hope to meet all the ones I have not seen, you all just keep growing.

Thanks Afrikan Yoga team in Africa. I want to thank Kwame Larbi, Kwame Hazel, (Afrikan Yoga, Ghana) for all your assistance, vision and tireless efforts in establishing Afrikan Yoga in Africa. Also Stephen Oddoye (Afrikan Yoga, Ghana) for his offering of 'Pharoahs' Guest House, Weija Accra as one of the homes of Afrikan Yoga. Thank you so much for your support.

Sawadago Bila Mohamed Tidiane 'Murari', Yogi and friend, even though you spent many years in Indian Ashrams as soon as you heard of Afrikan Yoga you immediately recognised it as your calling. This is a testament to all yogis of African descent in the Diaspora who still hold to the Indian system in spite of hearing about our rich cultural legacy. Thank you for raising the awareness of Afrikan Yoga in Togo, Benin and Burkina Faso. There is no doubt in my mind that more is to come from you my brother, as we work to bring Smai Afrikan Yoga back to our people.

Thanks to the Adornment Team; Margot and Sophia in particular, for your support at Brixton Art Space and showcasing Afrikan Yoga at Adornment events. May the ancestors bless you because you are truly amazing individuals.

I also want to thank Shamil Khan for the pictures of Sudras, Sidis and Dravidians.

To the students of my classes who humbly accepted my instructions and saw fit to nurture their bodies and spirit. With great joy and love I acknowledge you as my teachers in Smai. Thank you for your support without you my practice would have remained private and the healing genie would have not been released and shared. This book is a journey of love inspired by yourselves as you demanded it. You are my inspiration. Grow and teach higher consciousness. To all those who have graced my life though at times our relationship may be challenging, you give me food for thought, thank you.

Foreword

I was fortunate enough to be introduced to yoga almost thirty years ago (1979) and I began to practice immediately. The results were instant. I felt my body release, my mind relax and my energy and vitality levels increase. Yoga has completely transformed my life and for that I give thanks.

Over the years that I have practised, studied and taught yoga I have seen a steadily increasing number of people, all over the world, desire to re-connect with their spiritual essence; each person turning to yoga as the key that unlocks life's many mysteries.

The timeless wisdom of yoga reaches right back to the very first people who walked on our earth. The original cultures each had a tradition of Opening to Spirit and re-connecting to the very essence of our being. Today it is this longing in our souls that calls us to remember the ancient traditions.

Afrikan Yoga - Smai Taui is undergoing a powerful and timely resurrection. We are in the midst of what the Khemetic Dendera Zodiac calls the age of Hapi, the Aquarian age, thought to emerge between the years 2004-2012. This marks a time of major acceleration for the planet and her people. We are blessed with the potential of Hapi, who unites the higher and lower aspects of Self. This integration, this Smai, this union, this yoga expands and elevates consciousness.

Pablo Imani's book Afrikan Yoga, that propagates a system of healing and self-development with Afrikan origins for Afrikan people and those who feel an affinity with the practice, is long awaited. We give thanks to Pablo for answering his calling and offering you an opportunity to re-member, to re-connect and unite the disparate parts of yourself into a beauty-filled whole.

Let the pages speak to you, let spirit bless you and allow yourself to be transformed by the timeless teachings of Smai Taui.

C. Shola Arewa
Yoga Acharya (Master)
Author of Opening to Spirit

Preface

Yoga is on the rise and its popularity is due to the need to de-stress in an ever-growing stressful environment. There are countless amounts, of classes all over the UK. The British Wheel of Yoga, the largest yoga organization in the UK has a network of over 3,000 qualified registered teachers, not to mention many more that are registered with other organisations. I took up Chinese yoga commonly referred to as 'tai chi', to help alleviate my back problems. However, it was the practise of African yoga that healed my back pain within a week of steady practice. It proved to me that the system is a cultural practise, which is also directly linked to ones body type and that all healing systems are specifically created by and for the culture and the peoples' (body type) of that culture. More accurately termed 'Ethno medicine' in reference to *Dr Llaila O Afrika* and *Dr Jewel Pookrum.*

This also taught me that my genetic make up has a spiritual component that will grow or deplete with whatever I take on board as a spiritual path/practice.

Yoga has been taught to Afrikans by various Yogis who foundations are rooted in India. Yoga and its practices are no different to language, dress, food, or a cultural dance, for the language of Yoga today is Sanskrit which says to me if I do not blend with this language or call on (Mantra) Hare Krsna or Brahman etc then I am not a yogi. This lacks diversity of all peoples. I will go further and say that Yoga did not begin with Sanskrit because Afrikan people have Yogic practices that pre-dates the practices in India which where also founded by Afrikans. Even if one does not accept this fact I would like to present here a companion for those of African descent a very Ancient Yogic practice applied today. In present day and ancient yoga teachings the ultimate goal of yoga is union with the GODHEAD, Some masters have called this KRSNA in line with the Bhagavad-Gita, some have called it BRAHMAN in line with the Upanishads and some metaphysicians today call it CHRIST CONSCIOUSNESS.

Afrikans must also seek this aim in their own language and symbolism, in order to powerfully bring peace to this planet by first seeking it in themselves.

This book aims to address this with the use of our very own scriptures for example **'Coming Forth by Day', 'The Husia Sacred Wisdom of Ancient Egypt'** and various scriptures written by Nubians some of which compliment and predates the Hindu Buddhist texts. This is not to negate Taoist or Hindu text from which I have read and gained valuable food for thought and wisdom from. In this piece of work I have also applied **'The Sacred Wisdom of Tehuti'** to Afrikan Yoga and the principles found therein as well as offered a practical guide to Smai postures breath and meditation.

Introduction

The Reason why I am writing this book

There are several reasons why I have taken it upon myself to write this book. There is The Ancestors (Pa Neteru) who has guided me to this point, and I feel this strongly. I must mention that I have not taken this work or practise lightly. I have met death who has been friendly with me since childhood. Each time I have had to ponder on my existence and my purpose. The time when I got ambushed by 3 boys after school, I was around 11 or 12 years, we got in to a fight and they pulled my coat, which had a zipper that caught my throat but did not cut deep enough to slay me, then ran off while I laid there on the

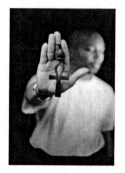

floor. I still have the scar today. The time, once again another fight, and I got pushed through a 2 storey window. I walked away with just a cut on my side by my kidneys. The time I had a gun put to my head by secret police in Cameroon, West Africa; I was able to talk my way out of that one and walk away. Then when I stood in front of an angry brother with a knife, saying he was going to stick me. I waited afraid that this was it and stood there ready to anticipate the thrust. It did not happen. A car crash on an autobahn (motorway) in Sweden, during a hip-hop tour where I was guest Dj, shook me up. I was not driving the van but we spun several times and hit the barricade without a pile up of cars that normally ensue on a busy autobahn; we all expected it but it did not happen and we were able to continue our journey dazed and thankful. Another car crash, and this time I was driving and it was a head-on collision. The car I was driving was completely written off, this time my children were in the backseat and I was able to climb out of the side window with just a few scratches and get them out. The paramedics said "someone up there loves you". The mechanic said "you are meant to be dead I've seen *man dead* for less". My 2 year old daughter had to have an emergency operation on her small intestine, because of the crash, or else she would have died. That took my acquaintance with death to another level. I began to hear the ancestors loud and clear. Now I got the message. I could no longer walk away from who I am and why I am here, my purpose. I could no longer live the same way that I have been living with the same mental approach. I had to die to be reborn. These series of experiences made me realise that life is precious and that purpose is essential to this earth plane.

There is of course my experience of smai tawi, sometimes spelt sema taui, or what many of you call yoga, which is a term I will use until Afrikans as whole are aware. I acknowledge that my initial introduction to yoga was not through a book, a guru or a need to have a good-looking healthy body.

I was fortunate to have two family cats in my home as a small boy. Growing up with cats, watching them stretch, observing their ability to deeply relax; purring in stillness and calmness, every muscle in a state of de-stress, yet they possessed so much agility and their running and hunting is second to none. I copied them just the same way our ancient ancestors studied various animals in order to develop their martial sciences. This experience and in-perience in childhood became a ritual.

However, it was only later when I understood the breath and the symbiotic relationship between animal and nature, man and Neteru, that this practice was more than just a few stretches to keep you supple.

At age 12 I attended a Muy Thai (Thai Boxing) class in Oldham, an area of Greater Manchester UK, where I grew up and was taught by Master Toddy a Master and Champion from Thailand. The attraction to Thai boxing I now find difficult to recall but ritual was a greater part of the training which at the time my Christian upbringing was causing me internal turmoil. Like many young men at that age I did not fully understand the spiritual nature of the training, with its incense, bowing, recitals, gold embroidery silky bright and colourful cushions, drums and cymbals. The hall where made to look like a Thai temple. I suppose my attraction at the time was the physicality of the training and the fierceness of the style, the violence that with my Christian upbringing I did not have a problem with. I often came out of training with cuts and bruises feeling jubilant that I gave someone a bloody nose or a black eye. In Thai I felt electric. Then at 14 I sustained an injury. I did not return to full contact training until I was 18. In the meantime I developed certain habits that martial and sport training gives you and that is stretching. I became a dancer in the clubs and surrounded myself with what is known as 'sugar foot people'

While stretching in public I recall in a theatre I was approached, by a tutor at the local dance school, to enrol and attend classes. Again I found myself at a cross roads as I wanted to be a book illustrator and move into graphic design as art was my passion. Art kept me out of trouble, not always but for the most part growing up it saved me from the older gangs of Oldham and Manchester. Even as a youngster at age 13-14 I had friends selling drugs and possessing guns; I had a fear of going down that road. I turned up for my dance audition, performed and was accepted at the school. However, I enrolled into Art school instead. At 21 I went onto college and University and gained a Degree in Visual Communication. During college I kept up dancing and stretching but not martial arts. In the summer holidays I would stay with my older brothers in London working and getting to know London. During such visits seeing me stretch and

11

my suppleness I was introduced to Hatha Yoga by my brother's girlfriend. I did not give it much thought as I thought it was just a nice way to enhance stretches I already knew. Yoga for me, like many of us Africans, spelt middle class, Hindu and white.

I drifted…

In 1993 a year after my graduation I had a fascination with Islam yet had strong connection with Mysticism of Africa and all things African. I would wonder in and out of Mosques searching for myself. In 1994 I met a brother from Islaamic Hebrews Holy Tabernacle Ministries. I read a scroll 'Sons of The Green Light' it spoke to my innerbeing as if it was an audio recording. For the next 2 years I studied the author of the scroll and his teachings in the library with note books, encyclopaedias, dictionaries, science books and any other reference books of relevance; without joining his organisation. I became a Sufi and would sit in Dikhr/Zikhr (Chanting) circles zikhring Allah and learning the art of meditation. The ecstasy of such chanting infused me with the oness of the Supreme.

I began experiencing visions, vivid dreams, and visitations of ancient and unexplainable beings, levitation and intense spiritual intuition. For some reason I felt called, chosen, what was their interest in me, why me?

In 1996 I joined and took my shahada. My teacher was known as Imam Isa who then became Rabboni Y'shua Bar El Hadi El Mahdi. I then joined the Ancient Mystic Order of Melchizidek a spiritual order. The emphasis was the awareness of self through culture and spiritual disciplines, we studied science, ancient histories and mythology, languages and etymology, esoteric science and three major world religions. These we not only studied we lived them Islam, Judaism and Christianity. In all that time from the age of 21 and starting University, I did not practise martial arts but I did keep on stretching. I would return to Martial Arts in the form of TaMuSet in 1996 introduced to me by my friend and brother Sean Lee (no relation to Bruce Lee well who knows) who's background is rooted in Wing Chung we sparred and played but most of our sessions involved the development of our Tepi Hesp (Aura) and sekhem (chi) spiritual spark, life force. We also spent a great deal of time exchanging information on Taoist philosophy which I had an interest that with my art took me to Japan where I visited Shinto Temples from time to time to meditate. In 1997 I travelled to see my spiritual master Amon Nubi Roakh Ptah who prior to meeting him in person, visited me in my dreams and schooled me in them. 1997 was a year of elation a year of intense highs and lows I was made homeless for the 2nd time in my life yet it was the year that I met my spiritual master for the first time. I then was introduced and encouraged to participate in Ka-zimba Ngoma by two friends Karumah also known as Ab Ankh Rem and Anwar a Zulu from Azania South Africa. Sean also encouraged me to attend the Ka-zimba Ngoma classes

12

at The Academy of Nubian Cultural Arts, London. Under the guidance of the Holy Tabernacle Ministries, (also known as HTM: Heliopolis, Thebes and Memphis) the spiritual and physical journey was now unfolding. In that same year, 2000 through a company called Codex my consort Ife organised the first visit to London of Dr Muata Ashby the famed Egyptian Yoga master whom now as authored over 30 books.

Dr Muata Ashby was already well known in the UK through his book Egyptian Yoga Vol. 1, which on meeting Ife I found she already had the book in her possession. I listened to his lectures with fascination and of course I took the experience of meeting Dr Ashby has an initiation into the philosophy and concept of yoga has an African creation. I studied several of his books and one in particular "The Movements of the Neteru", and practiced daily while studying Anatomy and Physiology. By the end of that year I was already a fully qualified and practising massage therapist bent on learning and applying Afrikan Healing principles. I learnt that Dr Muata Ashby was not the first to practise Afrikan style yoga in the U.S. There seem to be earlier exponents of the science such as a Brother called Khan, a Martial Artist and yogi, based in Houston. I was told by my mentor Dr Llaila O Afrika that Khan was the first to take the Afrikan approach to yoga in recent times in the states. Another teacher who has been teaching for the past twenty years is Yiser Hotep and apparently he was introduced to the practice of Afrikan yoga, by his teacher Asar Ra Hapi. Asar and Yirser have also developed a practical approach to yoga based on the spiritual aesthetics of the ancient Egyptians. However, Dr Muata Ashby was the first to write extensively on the subject of Egyptian Yoga, Yoga Philosophy, Mysticism and its African origins. His personality, writings, and teachings infused me with a self-belief. Years later I went on to discuss with him at further length the concept of Afrikan Yoga.

I noticed that the UK lagged behind as there were few African yogis and most if not all had devoted themselves to Indian yoga styles and had chose to teach those styles. I must mention Sister Shola Arewa who was for a while a lone teacher of Egyptian yoga. Shola was able to integrate Afrikan principles and made comparisons of Indian, Egyptian and Yoruba concepts to the chakras.

I ended up inheriting some of her students in my very first sessions!

One day while staying at a friend who is a devotee of Ausar Auset through the Ausar Auset Society in London. I was going through my usual stretching routine preparing for Ka-zimba training. The lady of the house and she is a true Het Heru being born in the month of Hathor said I was practising yoga. It then occurred to me that for the past 27 years of my life I had been practising some form of yoga. Over the phone I spoke to an old friend from college. "As long as I have known you, you've been practising yoga" he said. During our time at college he had a keen interest in yoga and later on he became a yoga teacher and sound healer.

But for me yoga was middle class Hindu and white. So what is this yoga that I'm doing and why am I doing it? This I will explain further down in this book.

The other reason is there is racism in the world of yoga that yes should not be there but it is. It has never been spoken about publicly until now.

"Follow the footsteps of your ancestors for the mind is trained through knowledge Behold their words endure in books. Open and read them and follow their wise counsel for one who is taught becomes skilled. Do not be evil for kindness is good. Make the memory of you last through the love of you".

The Book of Kheti, the Husia, Sacred Wisdom of Ancient Egypt

Yoga and Racism

The matter sometimes referred to as the 'race problem', is the basic-initial 'unfinished business', among people of the known universe. Therefore it is not possible to effectively speak and /or act to eliminate any major problem that involves people without first eliminating the problem of racism, in every area of activity, including economics, education, entertainment, labour, law, politics, religion, sex, and war.

In order to do this, it is necessary for victims of racism [non-white people], in effective numbers, to know and understand who the racist are, how they function, and for what ultimate purpose.

The victims of racism must also know and understand how the power of the racists (to practise racism) can be nullified and/or eliminated, by victims of racism, speaking and/ or acting as individual persons.

Neely Fuller Jr.

Racism is a cog in White Supremacy's machine. That means that there is a much bigger picture, to the experiencing of the bus driver not stopping for you at the bus stop or the subtle aggressive way you are treated in a restaurant, on the job or at school. Racism is prevalent everywhere the Education, Economic, Entertainment, Labour, Law, Politics, Religion, Sex, War and Science. It is a matrix, which we are all imbedded. The realisation of racism can be a painful experience. White supremacy is designed to make you feel hopeless and that there is no means of escape; encouraging you to just go long with the programme. The power we actually possess is our ability to create. This ability allows us to travel in our minds to realms through our melanin. We do not have to go along with the machine we can unplug and reconnect to being.

"The war between the man called the black man, the East Indian and the man called white; the pale man or European is not your war Nuwaubian[1].

It is a war between man and mankind. Yet you are deities, you are more than men. Their practices led to fear and intimidation, which in turn gave birth to another kind of worship-reincarnation, over exaggerated disciplines called Yoga and Patma Yoga, where one emulates deformed beings. Or piercing at the sun until they can no longer see, or fast until the poisons overcome their bodies, they call this foolishness perfection.

This is the mother of religious disciplines. What fools these mortals be.

They teach you to worship in fear of your deity, but not out of sincere love of your deities".

Holy Tablets Ch 3 Tablet 3: 176-178

The love and sincerity for our ancestors is our true form of yoga which is Tamare Smai Tawi, can be enacted and activated through Ari` Action Ankh Life Ka Spirit. In combination with the forces of TA earth, MA water, RE sun genes (the solar force) and our physical bodies using the science of breath Smai we can be healed.

When we reconnect to our former selves, through ritual, spiritual cleansing, meditation, chanting and the practise of Afrikan Yoga/Tamare SMAI, we are actually transcending the boundaries that are placed on us and are becoming a Neophyte of our culture awakening the sun genes (solar force) and switching on the coded purpose of the soul set 76 trillion years ago.

This reconnection is a serious and daily undertaking indeed a lifetime operation. The mere fact that you are reading this book implies that you are ready to break out of the boundaries placed on you as an Afrikan, and on you as a human being to engage in a new dimensional reality. The thought that yoga comes solely from India and can be only practised by Indians and Europeans under the many branches of yogic systems validated by Indian Swamis gurus is ridiculous. Africans have been practising what you call yoga FOR THOUSANDS OF YEARS IN AFRICA AND IN INDIA.

16. The cycle of births and deaths comes only through Jnana and perishes only through Jnana. Jnana alone was originally. It should be known as the only means (of salvation).

---

[1] This quote is not against Smai Afrikan Yoga it is a ref to the corruptions of the science. A Nuwaubian is a person who practices Wu-Nuwaupu. They can be of any race. They are also refered to as the Indigo children the guardians of the planet.

17-18(a). That is Jnana through which one cognises (in himself) the real nature of Kaivalya as the supreme seat, the stainless, the partless and of the nature of Sachchidananda without birth, existence and death and without motion and Jnana.

18(b)-19. Now I shall proceed to describe Yoga to you: Yoga is divided into many kinds on account of its actions: (viz.,)
Mantra-Yoga, Laya-Yoga, Hatha-Yoga and Raja-Yoga.

20. There are four states common to all these: (viz.,) Arambha, Ghata, Parichaya and Nishpatti.

21. O Brahma, I shall describe these to you. Listen attentively. One should practise the Mantra along with its Matrikas (proper intonations of the sounds) and others for a period of twelve years.

22. <u>Then he gradually obtains wisdom along with the Siddhis,(Blacks of India) (such as) Anima, etc. Persons of weak intellect who are the least qualified for Yoga practise this.</u>

23-24(a). The (second) Laya-Yoga tends towards the absorption of the Chitta and is described in myriads of ways; (one of which is) – one should contemplate upon the Lord who is without parts (even) while walking, sitting, sleeping, or eating. This is called Laya-Yoga.

24(b)-25. Now hear (the description of) Hatha-Yoga. This Yoga is said to possess (the following) eight subservients, Yama (forbearance), Niyama (religious observance), Asana (posture), Pranayama (suppression of breath), Pratyahara (subjugation of the senses), Dharana (concentration), Dhyana, the contemplation on Hari in the middle of the eyebrows and Samadhi that is the state of equality.

Yoga-Tattva Upanishad
Translated by K. Narayanasvami Aiyar

Question: *What about the Black colour?*

Shri Swamiji: *White and black - these are the main two. The white is bifurcated into seven colours. <u>Black stands opposite to white. White is pure consciousness, it represents Vidya-shakti, the highest spiritual power. Black stands opposite to white. Black is avidya, maya, ignorance or illusion. Avidya stands against knowledge. Black stands for avidya, white stands for vidya. In between come the</u>*

seven colours. White is the highest, black is the lowest and in between are those seven colours.

Quote From Chakras@shivayoga.net

These are highly respected teachers in the world of Yoga Swamiji is viewed as a saint in India yet these are his words in regards to the charkas which appear misguided handed down from an Aryan doctrine that absorbed the spiritual practises of the blacks in India and mangled it into racist teachings. How many times have we seen this non-scientific view of blackness and how different is this view from dictionaries written by Europeans? Black is more than a colour but a state of supreme balance and I will speak further on this in *Arushaats Connection to Melanin*

What must be understood is a system is in place that place the Afrikan on the lowest scale economically, politically socially, intellectually and this system is by design, even though according to European scientist you the Afrikan are the highest on the human scale, where the scientists rate you 6 and Europeans 1. These particular scientists actually called you hue man the man of colour and of blackness. *Ref: Vitamins & Minerals from A to Z by Jewel Pookrum/Afrikan Holistic Health by Dr Llaila O Afrika.* This 'White supremist system' and all other systems of control can be dismantled and it starts with your mind.

"It is said that what is called 'the spirit of an age' is something to which one cannot return. That this spirit gradually dissipates is due to the world's coming to an end. For this reason, although one would like to change today's world back to the spirit of one hundred years or more ago, [10,000 yrs or so ancient Afrika: authors note] *it cannot be done. Thus it is important to make the best out of every generation"*

Hagukure, The Book of the Samurai by Tsunemoto Yamamoto

The fact is that Afrikan Yoga speaks to us here and now and its science is that it can be applied where ever you are and no matter what age. We make the best of now. The time has come for us to develop new concepts out of our conditioning and to break the moulds that are no longer valid. Afrikan Yoga is for everyone and all can benefit from the forms, breath sciences and exercises (Hanu) giving them a strong healthy body and a positive mental outlook on life. However, the psycho spiritual levels of SMAI, chants *gaanun* and its hika in truth will greatly benefit at the deepest cellular/etheric level sun genes people, A free-Ka (ns) immensely. Afrikan Yoga has emerged to align you with your ancestors. Just as Hatha Yoga, Kali Yuga yoga, astram yoga, Iynegar or astanga yoga and the various other forms of yoga coming out of India aligns you with Hindu-Brahma ancestry. Of course you are told by those who practise and teach yoga that yoga will benefit everyone regardless of race, sex and class this is true in part but it is only a half-truth. Take for example most practitioners of yoga are women and most Gurus are men. Why? Remember Aryan culture is based on patriarchy and to this day women are told that they are not meant to practice yoga and why are all the movements and the mantras named and done in Sanskrit and not in Dravidian languages? Yoga is like most things that claim universality such as music, for example how many people you know who are non Chinese listen to Chinese music. Music transmits culture just like food, dance, clothing, language and yoga is no exception. It is my hope that Afrikan Yoga will be sought out has a healing practise by Afrikans as it is important that Afrikans heal themselves mentally, spiritually and physically in order to re-balance the planet.

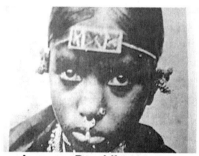

A young Dravidian woman

Castes and Division

We see confused states amongst us the world over and truly some of us are awakening out of these states. Those people who don't assist in the status quo by worshipping gods deities and demons representing the egotistical mind that are bent on keeping the planet in a wretched state.

This is also evident when looking at those who have taken on the Hindu religion and call themselves Hindus who in their former lives were Dravidians, Harrapans and other darker tribes of Indus Kush Ancient India, collectively named Shudras/sudras the people of the lowest cast existing in India today has for those who did not accept the system were labelled 'Untouchables'; The Outcaste.

"India's constitution not only does not interfere with cast, but fully upholds it". 'The Black Untouchables of India', V.T. Rajshekar African Presence in Early Asia.

The problem is: we do not see MAATian principles in everything.
The problem is: Yoga is mainly seen as just philosophy and not reality.
Philosophy is integral to the 5 P's system of control coming from the code of Hamurabbi, a Hindu in ancient Babylon, which is a pentagram of non-reality, utilising tricknology.

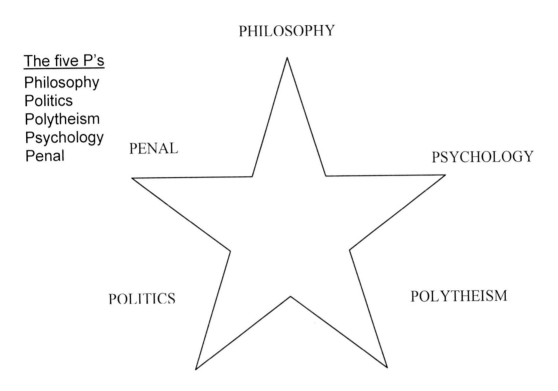

PHILOSOPHY

PENAL

PSYCHOLOGY

POLITICS

POLYTHEISM

The five P's
Philosophy
Politics
Polytheism
Psychology
Penal

"*The Aryan Brahmans professed that this system of human degradation was born from the God Brahma. They portrayed Brahma in human form, ascribing symbolic colours to the different regions of his body. The head of Brahma was white, reflecting the highest order of the caste, the Brahmanic or priest caste. The shoulders, arms, and torso of brahma were red, representing the kshatryias or warrior caste. The loins, hips and legs of Brahma were yellow, which identified the vaisyas or merchant caste, responsible for the economic sanctity of the empire. Last (and the least) were the black feet of Brahma, designating the unholy abode of India's blacks, upon whom the Aryan Brahma would eternally stand. From the pre-Vedic period onward, the title given to the original inhabitants is dasya or dasa, which means servant, and Sudra, which means slave*".

Wayne B Chandler, Ancient Future.

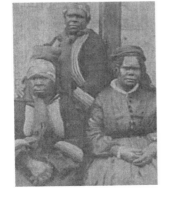

41. The works of Brahmins, Kshatriyas, Vaisyas and Sudras are different, in harmony with the three powers of their born nature.

42. The work of a Brahmin (priesthood caste) are peace; self-harmony, austerity and purity; loving-forgiveness and rightousness; vision and wisdom and faith.
43. These are the works of a Kshatriya (warrior caste): a heroic mind, inner fire, constancy, resourcefulness, courage in battle, generosity and noble leadership.
44. Trade, agriculture and the rearing of cattTe is the work of a Vaisya (merchant caste). And the work of a Sudra (slave caste) is service [slaving].

Bhagavad Gita 18.41-44

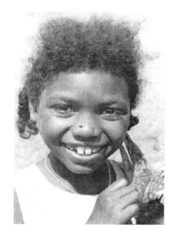

In the purushasukta hymn of the Rig-Veda there is a verse which says that of the primeval man 'Brahmin was the mouth, the Rajanya was as the arms, his thighs were the Vaishyas and from his Twi feet the shudra was born'.

N.K. Bose, The Structure of Hindu Society

In colonised India this way of looking at caste through the body of Brahmin was not only confined to human entities but to land, temples and all things were placed under this form of classification.

In the book 'The Structure of Hindu Society' also mentions the following…
"The social status of the different caste was determined by the yardstick of purity (Aryan) and impurity (non Aryan). Among the degraded caste, some were regarded as untouchable and some even unseenable".

This is also backed up by the laws of Manu the great 'law-giver' who the Vedic priest revered as the progenitor of the mankind son of Brahma by a incestuous relation with his own daughter.

The model of Manu was to be fiercely adhered to by all Aryan and those of Indo- European origin to maintain their racial consistency and status quo.

The Laws of Manu
1. He who weds a Sudra (Black) woman becomes an outcaste.
2. A brahmana who takes a Sudra to bed will sink into hell.
3. If a Sudra mentions the names of the caste of the Brahmans or Kshatriyas, an iron nail ten fingers long shall be thrust red of into his mouth.
4. If he arrogantly gives advice to the Brahmans, hot oil will be poured into his mouth and ears.
5. Food gets polluted by the smell of a pig, touch of a dog and the look of a Sudra.

6. If a Sudra hears the Vedas [the holy and religious texts of the Aryans], his ears shall be filled with molten lead. If he speaks them, his tongue will be cut out; and if he memorizes them, his body cut to pieces.
7. A Sudra must build his home outside the village, his wealth shall be dogs and donkeys and their dress shall be the garments of the dead, and they shall eat from broken dishes. Black iron shall be their ornaments, and they shall wander from place to place.[2]

This model of subjugation does not just sit in the continent of India but this is a global model of Aryan domination [Eurocentricism] where ever Afri-Ka (ns) are in the world.

There is racism in modern day yoga simply because modern day yoga has its legacy in Vedic traditions of the Brahmins. It is evident when no one bats an eyelid at the mention of Chinese Yoga, but when Afrikan Yoga is mentioned there are consternations, questions and disbelief.

The Process of Healing

People of Afrika "A free Ka" are led to believe that they did not originate anything. All that you see around you we had nothing to do with it. Often times I hear an Afrikan individual say well I can do yoga, Zen, Buddhism, Shinto and Celtic stuff because I'm universal. I am aware that we sometimes feel the need to be inclusive. Now is the time to pry your eyes open and view what scientist have already proven that all came from Afrika Tamare and the first world civilisations started in Afrika. So all these systems that we wish to be included in, are us anyway, right? So why are we not sticking to our thing or even trying to find out what our thing is? We have settled and submerged ourselves in a watered down warped and poisoned version of our ways of being. We have been bred out of our minds and out of our culture. We are led to partake of all other cultures appropriation of what Ethiopians Nubians Kushites Afrikans originated. This is discussed in more detail in the chapter on Yoga and Racism. Racism does exist yet we 'The modern day Afrikan' keep it in existence by our very thoughts and attitudes towards each other, our community and the world. We must realise that we should no longer be led by anyone.

---

[2] There are plenty of written and supporting documentation on the imbalances placed on the Afrikan the world over. However, the body of work by Neely Fuller Jr [the man who coined the term 'white supremacy']: The United Independent compensatory code/system/concept, a textbook/workbook for thought, speech and/or action for victims of racism (white supremacy), is a definitive in recognising and nullifying the effects of this social dis-ease.

We live on a day to day basis with a constant victim mentality. We are powerful enough to change the state of affairs in our lives and the affairs of this planet yet too many of us live in states of illusions. Our reality is re-created daily by what we think and how we think. We Afrikans can achieve what we will when we see and feel the joy of whom and what we are today as well as the pride of what we once were.

Now because I am pro-Afrikan does not mean I hate other races of people and I'm writing because I have an axe to grind, chip on my shoulder or just plainly ignorantly verbally abusing others. For those who are reading this book, this is not my intention. The abuse has got to stop and the healing must begin. This healing process often starts by facing what hurts and what appears to be discomforting so if you are European or Asian practitioner reading this book you too must heal and that is having an awareness of what your ancestors and peers and maybe you yourself are doing to the darker peoples of this world by not facing up to reality of your past and living off shame. Face that truth and develop your humanity to bring consciousness to this planet by working through Maat[1]. (Truth Justice Balance)

Let's work together for the sake of the planet and let the truth prevail. No more lies no more cover ups. Truth is Truth.

The Language in this book

Egypt had many dialects throughout its civilization. The dialects change over periods of time owing to the various invasions that eventually caused Egypt and indeed the entire African continent to decline. Some of these dialects are completely lost which is evident as Arabic is the main language of modern day Egypt. The language I used is called Nuwaupic as was introduced to me by my spiritual preceptor Amunnubi Ruakh Ptah this is the language not of the pharaohs or the general population but the language of Pa Neteru. A language whose origin was of the pre-dynastic period, that supposedly died out during the Greek and Roman invasions around 30BC and was replaced with Coptic. The western and European writers make claims that this old language was lost until a French man named Jean Francois Champollion deciphered the hieroglyphs in 1822. The claim is that he was the first to decipher the language correctly; this is a bold statement, as we now know that European translations of Afrikan languages and culture are not devoid of subjectivity and European cultural biase with its emphasis on entertainment value.

Would an Englishman accept a modern day African linguist deciphering old Anglo-Saxon or Germanic language and have that as the basis of their learning about that culture in that time for their school children?

This is not impossible however; we do have an option right now in regards to the Ancient language of Egypt and that is Amunnubi Ruakh Ptah a Sudanese by birth and linguistic speaker of 19 languages who reintroduced the lost language prior to the invasions called *Nuwaupic*. We also have several Afrikan melanated scholars around the world who have deciphered what is known as the '*Medu Neter*' sacred writings, for themselves and have a clearer insight as they do not use just intellect but genetic memory.

Nuwaupic

This language Nuwaupic appears also in ancient Sumer (Babylon) called to day Cuneiform. The cuneiform gave birth to Phoenician, Accadian, Chaldean, Ugaritic, Aramic, Hebraic and Syriac Ashuric Arabic. This is the language you will see and hear throughout this book. Nuwaupic can appear as script (language) or as a glyph (lanᴑuaᴑe). Nuwaupic is basically spoken in tones vibrating from the diaphragm which stimulate the spiritual seats in the body and is used to re-align human beings to The Guardians, *Pa Neteru*. I hope that Afrikan Yoga will be practised by Afrikans on the continent and around the globe using Afrikan languages that the individual is familiar with. Afrikan languages often use full vowel intonation and the diaphragm which is why Afrikans have deeper, melodic voices and the ability to sing the way they do. So all Afrikans can easily practice Smai science with the use of Xiosa, Twi, Ga, Fanti, Igbo, Zulu, Mende, Wolof, Fulani, Swahili etc., languages used presently. Nature's elements, Neteru, Orisha etc., remain the same for all of us.

As long as Afrikans begin to value what is theirs. We will take this (Smai-Afrikan Yoga) one of our many sciences back to where it belongs in our everyday *live-ity.*

Even though I have used the term Africa spelt purposely AfriKa or A Free Ka (a free spirit) on promotional materials and even to short cut the description of what I do to perspective students. I have chosen to redefine the word Africa as this word universally means a down trodden separated people and this piece of writing in no way wants to promote this present world view of Solar (sun) people. You may noticed that many are comfortable with this title Africa which derives from the Arabic word Farraq "to divide". The word Africa has been said to have various sources all of which are foreign to the present day 9 ether solar beings who reside on the Mother Father continent, at the centre of the world.

We as Ethiopians, Tamareans, Nubian Kushite peoples that means all 9 ether solar beings descended from an ancient and cosmic heritage.

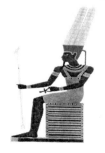

Af Re Ka is a definition that I explored as the Af is short for Aferti meaning Pharaoh. RE represents the sun specifically and The Most High and KA meaning spirit. We are truly sun peoples of a divine nature and are the descendants of Re. This is not myth this is by blood lineage as these beings 'The

Neteru' at one time walked this earth and that's why we have a genetic memory, restlessness, an affinity with nature; a deep love and compassion that only a 'being' of high culture could emanate. This is why we are so hard to destroy and this is why we are feared so much by those, who have a low level egotistic mind. This vague remenance of high culture is expandable; it can be nurtured and grown. The Neteru left us clues and guides having forseen their demise. That at some point we would lose our way, so we can find our way back. However, in the Yogic tradition the smai practitioner is a free spirited being and what Afrikans call for the world over is to be what we once were and that is to be free. We cannot be truly free unless we are free in body, mind and spirit. Afrikan Yoga frees the spirit by working through the body first. So A Free Ka (spirit) is the definition I use intermittently with Afrika. So do not look at this word merely as continent or place but see it as a state of mind and spirit.

"Lift up the self by the self, and don't let the self weaken, for the self is the self's only friend, and the self is the self's only foe".

The Grand Master Dr Malachi Z York
The Book of Urim and Thummim

TAMARE SMAI
Awakening Soul through
Earth Water & Fire union

One of the most difficult thing to do is to attempt to convince someone that what they have been led to believe all their lives is false. That the information that they have built their business on, or their leisure activities which they spent time and money over the years developing sentimental strings and even building their family unit is not only wrong but is more insidiously, a lie.

In reading this book I merely ask you to read with an open mind, take time to meditate and make the connection with your ancient Afrikan ancestors now miscalled Egyptians. They will provide you with the wisdom you seek in making the choices in regards to your health, your way of life "Ba Tarug" and the reconnection to the power source in which you are seeking.

"Truth alone is eternal and immutable; truth is the first blessing; but truth is not and cannot be on earth; everything has matter on it, clothed with a corporeal form subject to change, to alteration. The things of earth are but appearances and imitations of truth; they are what the picture is to reality".

Tehuti

24

Afrikan Yoga?

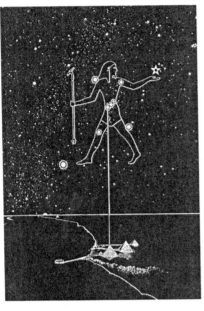

The word Yoga is derived from the Sanskrit root **'yuj'**, which means, union, join or bring together, taken from the Egyptian word **SMAI** which means union.

This union is symbolic of the divine principle within and without of us, our higher or real self. Yoga in the English word is yoke and in the Latin is **'yugum'** which when translated back to the English is 'married'. Now Sanskrit is an Indo Aryan language that was not spoken by the original inhabitants of India, known as Indus Kush in ancient times. Sanskrit was introduced to India around 1,500 BC.

Smai has been practised in Egypt North Africa for at least 5,000 B.C, and earlier in the greater part of Egypt, the Sudan, Ethiopia, Uganda etc.

The practise of SMAI was done by the Waab (priests) known in later times as Hery Heb (Teachers) and Sema (Funery Priests) of Ancient Egypt, which is seen as hieroglyphs, reliefs and statues dating thousands of years before any Indian guru or philosophies came into effect. Just has Kung Fu, Tai Chi and Chi gung are associated solely of Chinese and Chinese origin and not inventions and modifications based on earlier Kemetic Afrikan Schools. Yoga and India are interlinked in the minds of the world population as Indian origination. However, the practises associated with yoga started in Afrika.

"As a rule, Egypt is always treated differently from the rest of the world. No Egyptologist has ever dreamed that the ritual still exist under the disguise of both the Gnostic and canonical gospels, [yogic philosophy and practises] or that it was the fountain-head and source of all the books of wisdom claimed to be divine".
Gerald Massey, Egyptian Book of the Dead and the Mysteries of Amenta

The system and philosophies of yoga did not begin in India or by any of the Indians as you see them today. Not only that; the system of yoga that you see around today is a hybrid developed by the Brahmins sect, the priesthood of the lighter Indo Aryans who are of European stock and who invaded Indus Kush which is now known as India, a colony of Kush (Ancient Afrika). They also developed division on the Indian continent creating caste systems that degraded darker skinned peoples and religions in opposition to spiritual practices.

"In fact, all Chinese, Japanese and Hindu cultures and their forms of yoga, meditation, exercise, diagnosis, and treatments are biased in that they accentuate their own cultural frame of reference and disregard the African frame of reference"

Dr Llaila O Afrika, Afrikan Holistic Health

The various schools of Yoga include

Hatha (Het Heru) the best known school in the west, mainly but not exclusively physical.

Raja (Ra Ya) Yoga claims to be the highest yoga (Raja means "royal") but omits the physical. This yoga is used intermittingly with Astanga yoga another but more physical form of Hatha Yoga and derived from an Indian Brahmin Sri K. Pattabhi Jois.

Mantra (Ma NTR Ra) Japa and Nad Yoga concentrate on sound and meaning.

Swara (Shu Ra) Yoga on breathing.

Bhakti (Ba Akh Ta) Yoga objectives are placed on devotional prayer, meditation, and selfless love.

Karma (Ka R Ma) Yoga on work and service.

Kundalini (Anu/Ureaus) Yoga the raising of serpent or sekhem energy to integrate oneself with the higher consciousness (ANU)

Tantric (Ta NTR Ikh or Ta Nut Re) yoga attains enlightenment through the union and balance of male and female energy, either in sexual intercourse (Red Tantra or the left hand path) or in non-sexual (White Tantra or the right hand path); or in abstraction (Black Tantra Yoga where the practice is shamanic, which refers to energy sensitivity, earth energy and shape-shifting/alchemy).

Afrikan (A free Ka) Yoga/ Tama-re Smai contains all the above with concentration on ancestral linkage using them as examples of self-study and Haru/Heru as an example of self-mastery. Afrikan Yoga's ultimate goal is trancendance, union with nature, higher consciousness and the 'Most High'.

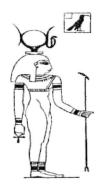

Hatha or Hat Hor

Hatha is said to be two words combined *'hat'* sun and *'ha'* moon. This not found in Sanskrit so this meaning must have had an older origin. The word Hatha has a further root stemming back to Huwa *"creative force of will"*

In part from the book Solar Biology or Lunar Astrology by Haru Hotep

*These eight elements were called Nu (Nawr) also called Nun (Nuwn) and Nunet (Naar), Heh (Huwa or **Hatha**) and Hehet (Hiya or Hathihi), Kek and Keket, the deities of darkness and void, who were responsible for removing the black dust cloud that covered the planet earth.*

Hatha derives from a principle or an action rather than a person and utilises what is called the eight limbs:
1. Yama – non-violence, truthfulness, chastity, avoidance of greed
2. Niyama – cleanliness of mind and body, devotion to God
3. Asanas, the conditioning of the body through the postures to train the mind to achieve meditation – stillness and ultimate peace.
4. Pranayama breathe control and the utilization of sekhem to energize the body and relax the mind.
5. Pratyahara – withdrawal of the senses and not to over indulge in the external world.
6. Dharana concentration on a subject for a short period of time this is often developed through the use of asanas/postures
7. Dyama – Meditation which comes from a developed dharana (concentration)
8. Samadhi – Deep Meditation this can be an outcome of all efforts combined to experience super/higher states of consciousness.

The modern day styles that are born out of Hatha Classical Yoga are Ashtanga Vinyasa, developed in Tibet and brought to the West by K. Pattabhi Jois Iyengar that is the study and emphasis on alignment developed in India and brought to the West by BKS Iyengar.

Power Yoga developed in America by Beryl Bender Birch with its emphasis on postures, the breath, heat, strength and internalisation specific for American mentality, and Dynamic Yoga developed in the UK by Godfrey Devereux both these are based on Ashtanga.

I am often asked: what is the difference between yoga (modern day yoga) and Afrikan Yoga (smai tawi ancient Kemitian/Egyptian yoga). The sanuy/posture seen in Afrikan yoga is numbered between 24 and 36. Where modern day yoga, that's what people mean when I am asked the difference is now said to have 840,000 postures.

Hatha Yoga

Hatha yoga of 1000 ACE original had very few postures and is not as ancient as many claim and the elaborate movements seen today is certainly not ancient.

We are aware of Hatha as Huwa creative force of will and its foundations in ancient Egypt (Afrika) as a science of intention and collaboration with the Neters through the use of breath and movement.

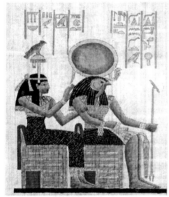

Het-Heru/.Hathor and Heru/Horus

Now for those of you who are aware of the meaning of the word Hatha have you ever wondered why the pronunciation of Hatha is *Ha-fa* instead of Hat (Sun) Ha (Moon)? Hatha is taken from Hathor, Het-Har or Het-Heru meaning *the dwelling place of Heru;* the sacred cow diety of ancient Egypt and also the consort of Heru. Hathor the wife of Heru gave birth to their son Har-smai tawy (Heru who unites the two lands). Hathor animal representation is the cow or *heifer*. The cow is well documented as the sacred animal of India and is worshipped as the symbol of a primordial mother.

In the Egyptian Prt M Heru, she is the one who urges the initiate to do battle with the monster Apep/Apothis. Apep in the mystical traditions is represented as the symbol of egoism that promotes thoughts, actions and evil, so as not to lose [his or her] heart, she cries out "take your armour". In a separate papyrus the initiate is told that she (Het-Heru) is the one "who will make your face perfect among the Neter and Netert, she will open your eye so that you may see everyday... she will make your legs able to walk with ease in the Netherworld, Her name is Het-Heru, Lady of Amenta". Het-Heru/Hathor represents beauty, joyousness, love and the bringer of happiness. Hathor is The Netert of the moon, the sky and the sun. A Netert of childbirth and young women, she is honoured as mother and is synonymous with Aset, they are often associated with each other and share the same attributes. Het-Heru represents the power of Re, the supreme spirit, therefore associating with her implies coming into contact with the boundless source of energy that sustains the universe. She is the joyful, happy side of Sakhmet, the fierce lioness who as the eye of Re, was an instrument of a destructive force and as the myth[3] goes began to slay man on earth to the point she got carried away and had to be subdued through the introduction of wine. Many European writers place emphasis on the wine aspect of the story, however, what is often missing in their writings is that Sakhmet as Hathor used dance, movement and hikau (song), *creative force* that brought cheerfulness and raised the heavy spirit. This is the saving of mankind. Hathor/Hatha uses the elements of movement, posture, hikau and positive mentality to subdue the destructive forces of the ego. Het-Heru/Hathor imbues potency and healing and there are still dances and rituals in honour of her in the Sudan today, known as the 'Sacred cow dances'. Contact with Het-Heru implies developing inner will power and vitality which engenders clarity of vision that will lead to the discovery of what is righteous and unrighteous (The practise of Afrikan Yoga/Tama-Re Smai)

Like everything else, life began with one thing in mind: to be and with this thought a thing became, and impregmentation existed, by the will of Huhi as Hu, ('the creative force of will), who gave rule of this side of the universe to Re, making him the highest order of **Sem.**

Sacred Records of Atum Re 1:205

Yoga today, which derived from Smai can be used as a means of reconnecting, present day Afrikans to our higher-selves the Neter/Orisha/Annunagi within and without. Smai/Yoga can be used to subdue the present destructive force within ourselves and our communities. This tool has lost its way through its Sanskrit meaning and now in the West has become quite beneficial yet of course like all *A Free Ka (n)* Afrikan origins through assimilation has lost its essence, its soul. The *Sanuyaat* sanuyaat postures explored in this book are on the walls in ancient Egypt. The various *'Hanuaat'* hanuaat movements of The Neteru and Pharaohs are here for us to switch on our Hui/Hu *creative force of will and transform again into Neters.*

---

[3] Wine is merely symbolic of the intoxicating feeling of the oness with the supreme through *'the creative force of will'* Hu.

The Earliest Known Inhabitants of India...
The Harappan

The Harappan civilization spreads all over India; 1,000 sites have been uncovered by archaeologists; the two main cities being Mohenjo-Daro and Harappa dating as far back as 3000 B.C.

The Harappans flourished along the river 'Indus' as did the Sumerians along the Tigris Euphrates and the Khemitians along the Nile.

The Harappans farmed and cultivated cotton. They had their own script and even though they were mainly pastoralist they were also builders who had drainage and sewage systems in their homes and throughout their settlements. The Harappans even formed bodily decorations using beads, copper, silver, gold and bronze to form necklaces and bangles.

The Harappans have been favoured by scholars to be the earliest inhabitants of India and often seem to be used as a description of the Dravidians even European and Indian scholars find them to be Black and Africoid

Those of us who have looked very closely at India's population, history and culture find India to be very mixed.

"In India… there are also traces of intermingling with the Negro race to which part of the darkness of the skin so widely prevalent in India may be attributed".
Elliot Smith, Human History, pp. 134-145 London, 1934

Marco Polo described the inhabitants of India as black and adorned with massive gold bracelets and strings of rare and precious gems. They had temples and priests. Vasco de Gama while circumnavigating the globe found the inhabitants black. (From the book: The Wonderful Etheiopians of the Ancient Cushite Empire, Chapter 15, The Civilization of India)

30

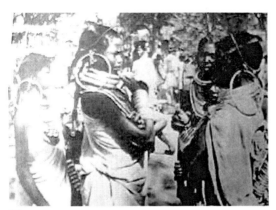

Harrapans

The people about whom I have been speaking of are descendents of Cushites they are a combination of two Black races, the Black Negroid (resembling Africans) and the Black Australoid (resembling Australian Aborigines. India is known to have some of the purest Black people on earth. These include the Black Dalit/Untouchables who were kept segregated and isolated for thousands of years by the 'Indo-Europeans", who invaded India from North-Eastern Europe. The brown-skinned to fair skinned people with features similar to Middle Eastern and Iranian people are of Caucasian origins and live mainly in the North West of India.

The Ethiopian Dravidians

The Dravidians in ethnic type are Ethiopian and are the race of India from which her civilization originated. Megathenes said that the natives of India and Ethiopia were not much different in complexion or feature. Dravidians are short like the race of the Mediterranean called Iberians and the Chaldeans. Their complexions are black or very dark. Their hair is plentiful and crispy. Their heads are elongated with the nose very broad. They occupy the oldest geological formation of India. They are descendants of that race of black men with short woolly hair that were the primitive inhabitants of ancient Media, Susiana and Persia, mentioned repeatedly in the Iranian legends, and whose faces look out at us from the sculptures of Babylon and Nineveh. Dravidian is spoken by forty-six millions of India, not including the numerous uncultivated hill tribes and retired communities. A form of speech similar to it is spoken in Beluchistan, which originally was Kushite.

Concept of the Dravidian Race

The identification of the Dravidian people as a separate race arose from the realization by 19th-century Western scholars that there existed a group of languages spoken by people in the south of India, which were completely unrelated to the Indo-Aryan languages prevalent in the north of the country. Because of this, it was supposed that the generally darker-skinned Dravidian speakers constituted a genetically distinct race. This notion corresponded to European belief of the time, according to which darker-skinned peoples were more "primitive" than the light-skinned whites. Accordingly, Dravidians were envisaged as primitive early inhabitants of India who had been partially displaced and subordinated by Aryans. The term Dravidian is taken from the Sanskrit "drÇvida", meaning "Southern". It was adopted following the publication of Robert Caldwell's *Comparative grammar of the Dravidian or South-Indian family of languages* (1856); a publication which established the language grouping as one of the major language groups of the world.

http://en.wikepedia.org

Speaking of languages, this is what Clyde A. Winter said in his researched piece called the 'Cultural Unity of African languages':

Dravidian languages are predominately spoken in southern India and Sri Lanka. There are around 125 million Dravidian speakers. These languages are genetically related to African languages. The Dravidians are remnants of the ancient Black population who occupied most of ancient Asia and Europe.

32

Clyde further informs us of the unity between Ancient Indian languages and African languages by making cultural and linguistic comparisons. The Dravidians have maintained their ancient African Heritage. There are numerous affinities between Dravidian and Black African culture and languages. As in Africa the Dravidians built there both small and large vessels from a single log or planks tied together. This method of boat construction has been common in Africa since the rise of ancient Egypt, and continues today in East Africa, Chad and along the Niger River. In both Africa and Dravidian India the people were organized into various "caste" or corporations. Many of the corporations such as that of the blacksmiths in Africa and India have corresponding names e.g., Wolof Kamara and Telugu Kamara. There are similarities in agricultural technique in Africa and India. For example, both groups used the hoe for tilling the ground, manuring the ground to fertilize crops, terracing irrigation and canal building. There are also affinities in animal husbandry, and even the names of animals. For example, sheep: Wolof xar, Brahui (Dravidian) xar 'ram'; and cow: Wolof nag, Serere nak, Tamil naku 'a female buffalo' and Tulu naku 'heifer'. There are also similarities between the Dravidian and African religions. For example, both groups held a common interest in the cult of the Serpent (*Kundalini*) and believed in a Supreme God, who lived in a place of peace and tranquility. There are also affinities between the names of many gods including Amun/Amma and Murugan. Murugan, the Dravidian god of the mountains, parallels a common god in East Africa worshipped by 25 ethnic groups called Murungu, the god who resides in the mountains. In addition among the Ali tiravitar, the system of inheritance passes from the uncle to his nephews, instead of to his sons (maru makkal Tayam) as in Africa. And in both South India and the Western Sudan of Africa, the dead were buried in terra cotta jars.

Unity between Afrikan and Ancient Indian (Dravidian) Languages

Below Clyde Winters provided linguistic examples from many different African Supersets (Families) including the Mande and Niger-Congo groups to prove the analogy between Dravidian and Black African languages.

Linguistic evidence for Indo-African linguistic unity

Many scholars have recognized the linguistic unity of Black African (BA) and Dravidian (Dr.) languages. These affinities are found not only in the modern African languages but also that of ancient Egypt. These scholars have made it clear that lexical, morphological and phonetic unity exist between African languages in West and North Africa as well as the Bantu group.[4]

Dravidian languages are predominately spoken in southern India and Sri Lanka. There are around 125 million Dravidian speakers. These languages are genetically related to African languages. The Dravidians are therefore remnants of the ancient Black population who occupied most of ancient Asia and Europe.

K.P. Arvaanan (1976) has noted that there are ten common elements shared by BA languages and the Dr. group.
They are (1) simple set of five basic vowels with short-long consonants;
(2) vowel harmony; (3) absence of initial clusters of consonants; (4) abundance of geminated consonants; (5) distinction of inclusive and exclusive pronouns in first person plural; (6) absence of degrees of comparison for adjectives and adverbs as distinct morphological categories; (7) consonant alternation on nominal increments noticed by different classes; (8) distinction of completed action among verbal paradigms as against specific tense distinction; (9) two separate sets of paradigms for declarative and negative forms of verbs; and (l0) use of reduplication for emphasis.

---

[4] The Bantu group, see Dr Ben Jochannan

There has been a long development in the recognition of the linguistic unity of African and Dravidian languages. The first scholar to document this fact was the French linguist L.Homburger (1950, 1951, 1957, and 1964). Prof. Homburger who is best known for her research into African languages was convinced that the Dravidian languages explained the morphology of the Senegalese group particularly the Serere, Fulani group. She was also convinced that the kinship existed between Kannanda and the Bantu languages, and Telugu and the Mande group.

Dr. L.Homburger is credited with the discovery for the first time of phonetic, morphological and lexical parallels between Bantu and Dravidians. For example, she noted that the Bantu infinitive with a final -a, the subjunctive in -e, the preterit in -i or -idi, and the doer's name in -i, are all found with identical values in Kannanda and other Dravidian languages. Dr. Homburger also found that both the Bantu languages and Kannanda there was the causal suffix -is.

Prof. Tuttle (1932) also contributed to the investigation of links between African and Dravidian languages. In a short paper he wrote in the 1930"s he presents numerous lexical and grammatical parallels for Dravidian and the Nubian.

One of the most interesting studies done to date on the links between African and Dravidian languages was the work of N. Lahovary (1963).

Professor Lahovary in his review of the possible link between the languages spoken by the founders of the major ancient civilizations gives a stimulating discussion of cognates among various African languages and Dravidian (Dr.). He gives numerous lexical examples for the ancient kinship of the Dravidian group and BA – (Black African) languages, including ancient Egyptian, Hausa, Bantu, Nubian and Somali, to name a few.

As a result of the linguistic evidence the Congolese linguist Th. Obenga suggested that there was an Indo-African group of related languages. To prove this point we will discuss the numerous examples of phonetic, morphological and lexical parallels between the Dravidian group: Tamil (Ta.), Malayalam (Mal.), Kannanda/Kanarese (Ka.), Tulu (Tu.), Kui-Gondi, Telugu (Tel.) and Brahui; and Black African languages: Manding (Man.), Egyptian (E.), and Senegalese (Sn.)

COMMON INDO-AFRICAN TERMS

ENGLISH	DRAVIDIAN	SENEGALESE	MANDING
Mother	Amma	Ama, Meen	Ma
Father	Appan,	Abba Ampa,	Baaba Ba
Pregnancy	Basaru	Biir	Bara
Skin	Uri Nguru,	Guri	Guru
Blood	Nettaru[5]	Deret	Dyeri
King	Mannan	Maansa, Omaad	Mansa
Grand	Biira	Buur	Ba
Saliva	Tuppal	Tuudde	Tu
Cultivate	Bey	Mbey	Be
Boat	Kulam	Gaal	Kulu
Feather	Sooge	Siige Si,	Sigi
Mountain	Kunru	Tuud	Kuru
Rock	Kallu	Xeer	Kulu
Stream	Kolli	Kal	Koli

. . . . .PRONOMINAL PARALLELS IN BA AND

VOWEL SYSTEM OF DRAVIDIAN
BLACK AFRICAN
 i u ii uu
e o ee oo
a aa

2. Ancient Egyptian and Dravidian. There are numerous corresponding lexical items in Egyptian and Dravidian languages, below are a few:

Language	abscess	abyss	to go with	build
Egyptian	bnw	t kiki	hp hr	qd
Dravidian	pun	kedu	po -nnu	kattu

----

[5] Nettaru=blood Dr Malachi Z York often spoke about the blood link between the Neteru and Afrikans today. It is through the blood and bone marrow that Ancestors genes are in encoded. In Afrikan Yoga we meditate on the flow of blood and the bones in postures and movements.

Language	chief great/noble	young	house
Egyptian	neb bw	hrd	I
Dravidian	nab'grand' bal	kura il,	II

Language	speak	small	to be
Egyptian	mdw sr,	srr	wnn
Dravidian	matu	siru	unn-

Nubian and Dravidian cognates

English	Dravidian	Nubian
play	aad	od
sister	akka	keg
say	an,	en onul
woman, daughter	asa	as
elephant	ane,	enugu onul
bean	avari	ogod
water	er	iri
mother	ia	een
to be	ir	in
true	olle	ale
day	ulla	ul
son	maga	ga
mountain	male	mule
fish	min	anissi
eat	tin,	ti di
stone, rock	kal	kulu
tongue	na nar,	nad
shore	kare	gaar

The evidence is clear that the Dravidian and Black African languages should be classed in a family called Indo- African as suggested by Th. Obenga. This data further supports the archaeological evidence accumulated by Dr. B.B Lal (1963), which proved that the Dravidians originated in the Fertile African Crescent.

Thundy believes that the Dravidians may have left Nubia after Senefru (c.2613 B.C. conquered Nubia. Senefru's raid caused much destruction and may have encouraged many Kushites to flee Nubia for safe areas of settlement.

Calumet testifies that from ancient accounts and from all recent research, culture and civilization spread into Egypt from the south and especially from Meroe. Egypt, ruled at first by several contemporary kings, was finally united into one great kingdom. Priesthood seemed to have governed the land. The head of the state was a priest. The sacred books of the Hindu speak of an "Old Race",(Tarites, Twa and the Nubuns ancestors to the Nuwaubians/Tamareans/Kemetians Ancient Afrikans) that came down from Upper Egypt and peopled the delta. They mentioned the Mountains of the Moon and the Nile flowing through Barabra. Herodotus says in his Second Book, "They say that in the time of Menes/Narmer (first Dynasty) all Egypt except the district of Thebes was a morass, and that no part of the land now existing below Lake Myris was then above water. To this place from the sea is seven days passage up the river". Diodorus Siculus (*Author of Library of world history*) says in Book Three, "The Ethiopians say that the Egyptians are a colony drawn out of them by Osiris; and that Egypt was formerly no part of the continent but a sea at the beginning of the world, and that it was afterwards made land by the river Nile".

Upper Ancient Egypt

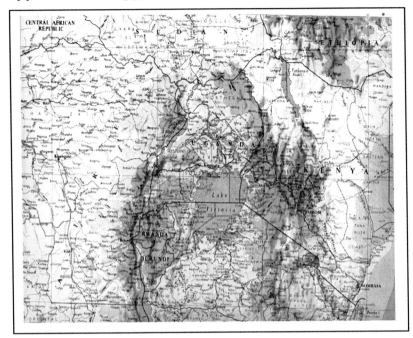

Lower Ancient Egypt.

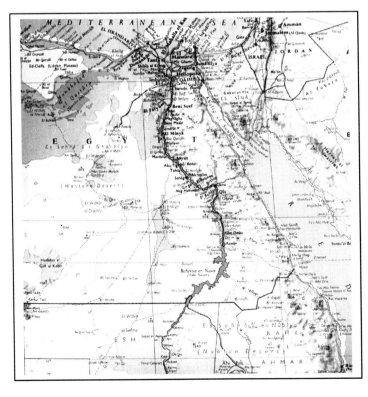

Ancient Egypt/Khemet spread from the North of present day Afrika down to Kenya, Uganda and Zimbabwe.

Egyptians are not exclusively north Afrikans. The original Egyptians of today live all over the world. We reside in the south and in the west as well as the entire Diaspora. The original culture of Egypt came from what was called Upper Egypt at the origin of the Nile, Uganda on through Kenya, and the Congo where the Twa or Pthar-ites reside and this culture spread throughout all of Afrika and indeed on to other parts of the world.

The All is I am

"I am the Universe and the Universe is I

I am balanced, graceful and beautiful.

The Universe is balanced, graceful and beautiful.

I am the Universe and the Universe is I".

Khonsu Sekhem Ptah

The Foundations of Afrikan Yoga

Firstly we have to deal with the word **TA** t a in TAMARE a name many of us call our children sometimes pronounced and spelt Tamara or Tamerri. Ta is earth and is the grounding foundation of the aspirant. Ta earth is the first stages of the practise of Tamare Smai sanuyaat (forms). This principle is to keep your feet firmly on the ground while exploring the god-head of Re. Ptah the Ancient Deity of Kemet father of Ra/Re is the being through the manifestation of thought and tone set the motion of creation through HuHi.

Ptah used the sound Aum, used by the Mystics and spiritual aspirants today to stimulate higher senses, visualisation and healing. Ptah is the being known to be the Deity of physical creation; the creator of matter.

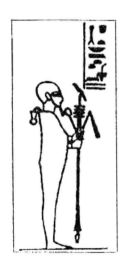

Ptah pronounced Tar. The earliest of the ancient names of Egypt is Tar ("Black as tar" comes to mind when speaking of the Tarites)

The word Pygmy or should I say an insulting name calling of the Ancient peoples of Afrika who's true name[6] is Ptahrites or Tarites where your pre-history pre-dynastic people of Ancient Khemet KMT known as TA MA RE, who where indigenous to the planet. They studied or knowing how to manipulate the elements through the mind soul and spirit. They were remembered and defied just how Michael Jordon, Pele, Muhammad Ali, or Billie Holiday his honoured today. The elements and principles began to have a face and name in remembrance of these great masters and in turn we found inspiration and a connection through a blood-

---

[6] **Note**: However through out time we are known and called by many names and what you chose to call yourself must have a connection to your culture, land, dress, customs and laws that ultimately reflect all the above. Black by modern day definition has no culture etc and appears to be just a colour, this too is an illusion.

41

link, a genetic re-coding which on further inspection leads in to atoms back to the un-manifested back to the source. This is one of our many tools of connectivity.

The Deity Ptah pronounced Tar, whose wife was Sekhmet and his son Neferten (or Nefertem/Nefertum), made up the Memphite triad or Trinity.

Ptah was associated with Hephasteus by the Greeks, and as he was the deity of Blacksmiths the Romans called him Vulcan after their own God of the forge.

Ptah invented the methods and techniques of the craftsman and was the deity of Masons his High priests held the title 'Master Builder' or 'Supreme Leader of Craftsmen'. This forging done by the original blacksmiths was the forging of the internal and eternal soul, the transformational development of ones character.

The Ptarhites where small people about 4ft tall yet they where mental giants. Note. He was an earth deity and had links with the underworld

Secondly the word **Ma ma** derives for Tamarean Nuwaupic word ma or mu for water and is also the first two letters in Ma'at.

Ma'at is the ancient one who represents the symbol of truth, justice and world order, and is the female deity of weighing the Ab "heart". Ma'at always wears the ostrich feather a symbol of law, truth, right and justice. The word Ma'at means "that which is straight, right, true, sincere and honest *and perhaps even Tao or* Balance". She is the woman of the judgement hall; her feather was balanced against the heart of the deceased to determine whether he had led a pure and honest life. Ma'at was represented as a tall woman with an ostrich feather in her hair. Ma'at is the wife of Tehuti, Djehuti, Zehuti, (Thoth) and the Daughter of Re. Ma'at assisted Ptah, (Ta) and Khnum in carrying out rightly the work of creation order by Tehuti. She is the order that rules the world through balance.

Ma'at symbol the ostrich feather is also the quill and the hand symbol Yod, or Y which is the letter I (I and Y are interchangeable in the old languages) As in I and I or the I in Egipt. I being the 9th letter of the alphabet. 9 being the highest number 9 to 9th power. Nine mind etc... The use of the hand was adapted by the monotheist and became the hand of God, Allah or Jehovah. The ostrich feather was used as a pen for writing the hieratic script of Ta-Mara, Tama-re, it became the beak of the Ibis bird for the Deity Tehuti which symbolised the scribe that wrote the law of the Torah, your bible and it gave birth to the Qu'ran (Koran), all from the Egiptians, which their God Yahweh was suppose to have written by hand, for the Haribu-aat (Hebrews), they show the symbol of the extended finger, which is the beak of the Ibis bird, under Mose , who became Moses, Mosheh and Muwsa. All from the Egiptian Mose meaning "child" of the school of Thothmose who was a student of Thoth, Tehuti who became Hermes, from the latin

Hermeticus, meaning "alchemical" borrowed by the Greeks and used as a god, son of Zeus and Maia.

In the words of The Master Teacher Amun Nubi Roakh Ptah, ***"Ma'at is the pillar of justice and is the spiritual struggle against injustice. We the Tama-reans, (Afrikans) must learn to assimilate, to distribute and to pass judgment justly and with impartiality. We must stand for true Ma'at,*** *"that which is right".*

The declarations of Ma'at known as the 42 declarations of innocence are the principle basis of the Ten Commandments. To call them negative confessions is a subtle aggressive ploy by some Europeans to place in the minds of Afrikans that there is something wrong in declaring the principles that we should live by.

By conservative estimate, the 42 Oracular Principles of Maat (Declarations of Innocence) were written approximately 1,500 years before the writing of the Ten Commandments. By comparing the two documents, one will find striking similarities. The 42 Oracular Principles of MAAT are drawn from the A free ka (n) Holy book Pert m Hru, (Book of Coming Forth by Day), the worlds oldest book of Holy scriptures. With these laws, our Ancient Ancestors maintained a society without a police force for thousands of years. In the early morning say "I will not", and in the evening say "I have not.". This is how we perform a moral inventory.

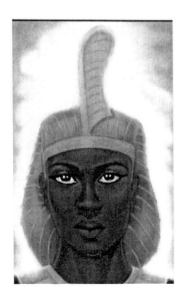

Neter Naat

Netert Maat

Baka (Morning declaration)

THE 42 ORACULAR PRINCIPLES OF MAAT
(PRT M HRU)

1. I **Will Not** do wrong
2. I **Will Not** Steal, rob. Cheat
3. I **Will Not** act with violence (brutalize)
4. I **Will Not** kill (cause murder for sport)
5. I **Will Not** be unjust (biased)
6. I **Will Not** cause pain (inflict cruelty, torture or needless injury)
7. I **Will Not** waste food or squander resources
8. I **Will Not** lie (perjure)
9. I **Will Not** desecrate holy places (be irreverent)
10. I **Will Not** speak evil.
11. I **Will Not** abuse my sexuality
12. I **Will Not** cause the shedding of tears
13. I **Will Not** sew seeds of regret
14. I **Will Not** be an aggressor
15. I **Will Not** act guilefully
16. I **Will Not** lay waste the plowed land
17. I **Will Not** bear false witness
18. I **Will Not** set my mouth in motion against any person
19. I **Will Not** be wrathful or angry except for a just cause
20. I **Will Not** copulate with a man-wife or woman-husband
21. I**Will Not** desecrate the wife of a man or husband of a woman (commit adultery)
22. I **Will Not** pollute myself (my body temple)
23. I **Will Not** cause terror
24. I **Will Not** pollute the earth
25. I **Will Not** speak in anger
26. I **Will Not** turn from the words of right and truth (disobedience to ones conscience)
27. I **Will Not** utter curses (debase my power of speech)
28. I **Will Not** initiate a quarrel (instigate disharmony)
29. I **Will Not** be excitable or contentious (impatient)
30. I **Will Not** prejudge (be presumptuous)
31. I **Will Not** be an eavesdropper
32. I **Will Not** speak over much

33. I **Will Not** commit treason against the ancestors
34. I **Will Not** waste water
35. I **Will Not** do evil
36. I **Will Not** be arrogant (insolent)
37. I **Will Not** blaspheme NTR (The Most High Mother-Father of Creation)
38. I **Will Not** commit fraud
39. I **Will Not** defraud Temple offerings
40. I **Will Not** plunder the dead (grave robbery, piracy)
41. I **Will Not** mistreat/abuse children.
42. I **Will Not** mistreat/abuse animals.

In the shadow hours we will repeat the 42 replacing 'I will not' with 'I have not'.

Ushat (shadow/night declaration)

THE 42 ORACULAR PRINCIPLES OF MAAT
(PRT M HRU)

1. I **Have Not** done wrong
2. I **Have Not** Stole, robbed or Cheat
3. I **Have Not** acted with violence (brutalize)
4. I **Have Not** killed (cause murder for sport)
5. I **Have Not** been unjust (biased)
6. I **Have Not** cause pain (inflict cruelty, torture or needless injury)
7. I **Have Not** wasted food or squander resources
8. I **Have Not** lied (perjure)
9. I **Have Not** desecrated holy places (be irreverent)
10. I **Have Not** spoken evil.
11. I **Have Not** abused my sexuality
12. I **Have Not** caused the shedding of tears
13. I **Have Not** sewn seeds of regret
14. I **Have Not** been an aggressor
15. I **Have Not** acted guilefully
16. I **Have Not** laid waste the plowed land
17. I **Have Not** bear false witness
18. I **Have Not** set my mouth in motion against any person
19. I **Have Not** been wrathful or angry except for a just cause
20. I **Have Not** copulate with a man-wife or woman-husband
21. I **Have Not** desecrated the wife of a man or husband of a woman (commit

adultery)

22. I **Have Not** polluted myself (my body temple)
23. I **Have Not** caused terror
24. I **have Not** polluted the earth
25. I **have Not** spoken in anger
26. I **have Not** turned from the words of right and truth (disobedience to ones conscience)
27. I **Have Not** uttered curses (debase my power of speech)
28. I **Have Not** initiated a quarrel (instigate disharmony)
29. I **Have Not** be excitable or contentious (impatient)
30. I **Have Not** prejudged (be presumptuous)
31. I **Have Not** be an eavesdropper
32. I **Have Not** spoken over much
33. I **Have Not** committed treason against the ancestors
34. I **Have Not** wasted water
35. I **Have Not** done evil
36. I **Have Not** been arrogant (insolent)
37. I **Have Not** blasphemed NTR (The Most High Mother-Father of Creation)
38. I **Have Not** committed fraud
39. I **Have Not** defraud Temple offerings
40. I **Have Not** plundered the dead (grave robbery, piracy)
41. I **Have Not** mistreated/abused children.
42. I **Have Not** mistreated/abused animals.

The ten Virtues of the initiates under the guidance of Ma'at

1. **Control your thoughts**
2. **Control your actions**
3. **Have devotion and purpose**
4. **Have faith in your masters ability to lead you along the path of truth**
5. **Have faith in your own ability to accept truth**
6. **Have faith in your ability to act with wisdom**
7. **Be free from resentment under the experience of persecution**
8. **Be free from resentment under experience of wrong**
9. **Learn how to distinguish right and wrong**
10. **Learn to distinguish the real from the unreal**

Ma ma

The principle of water is of a feminine nature and utilises patience perseverance and creative energies in order to grow and nurture seeds. We may only look at a few ancestral deities of water to clearly understand water principles.

The Diety Tefnut is moisture and represented in the "*Hanu-aat*" movements, "*Hudu*" Afrikan Tai Chi and "*Ragus*" dance of Afrikan Yoga/Tama-re Smai.

The word Ma ma is water, which symbolises the womb, or the embryonic sac that the fetus rests in before leaving the womb, it's the primordial water.

Sacred Records of Atum Re (scroll 1.129)

The Afrikan cosmology of the 8 Rashunaats also known as the Khemenu (8), Ogdoads

These beings are known as the primordial ancestors or the Adams and Eves, which represents periods of time in our evolution and is often noted by European writers as tadpoles, reptilians and frogs that is why the word evolution is apt as they are the symbolic development of growth throughout time and also within the womb of our mother. Ever wonder why in our English school they made you do experiments on frogs in biology class, this is because a frog layed out is close to the human anatomy.

The first set
Nun Nunet

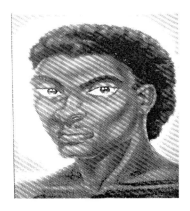 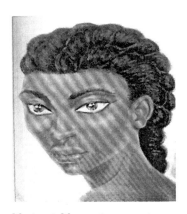

Neter Nun nun   **Netert Nunet** nunet

They are the first stage of our evolved state; the sea-men and the first period of gestation. Nun is the male part meaning 'deep abyss' 'chaos' and Nunet is the female consort meaning 'The abyss'. They are the deities of water. 3/4ths of the human body is water and the lymphatic and circulatory systems are the source of life and reproduction, water is the most important element in existence and a needed source of conduction.

The second set
Heh Hehet

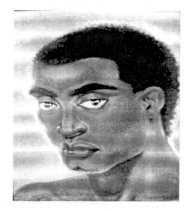
Neter Heh heh

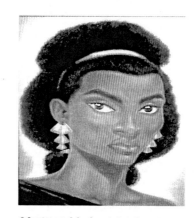
Netert Hehet hehet

The second set of our evolution. Is represented by the male Neter Heh 'infinity' and his female consort Netert Hehet 'eternity' They were also known as the deities of immeasurable time they were represented by tadpoles.

The third set
Khek Kheket

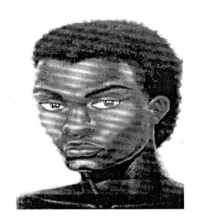

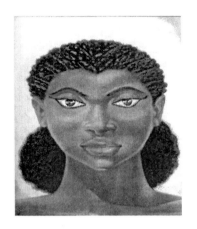

Neter Kek kek

Netert keket keket

The third state of our evolution is Neter Kek male deity of Supreme darkness and Netert Keket female deity of Supreme darkness.

The fourth set
Amun Amunet

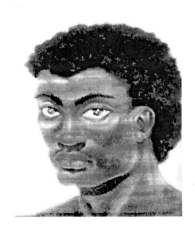

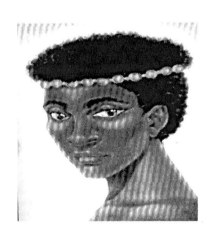

Neter Amun amun

Netert Amunet amunet

Amun 'the hidden one' is the male part and Amunet 'she who is hidden' the female consort. They are the deities that bred on earth and are the earth deities or our very first Adams and Eve, Human beings who breathed.

The first three were your original water beings and show our basic stages of evolution that is played out through 9 months of pregnancy. That follows our watery beginnings into breathing Adams coming out of the darkness of the womb. Our ancient Afrikan scientists are well aware of this and symbolised them through our many stories of creation.

Maybe we should rename this planet H2o because it has far more water on it than earth and all the water is connected from the rivers to the streams to the oceans to even the clouds. The continents sit on top of the water and have been drifting since the pre-Cambrian age. This is an aquarium for there is water in the air and absolutely everything else on this planet. From your rocks to your plastics will some how contains water and our bodies are made up of over 70% of the substance, we would absolutely shrivel and die with out it. Our skins would peel and flake like reptiles if we did not submerge ourselves in water every day.

Water is fundamental and we need to take it keep our selves in a state of good health and of course social inclusion.

Drew Fobbester online nutritionist says **"if you want well moisturised skin, hydrate. If you did nothing else but drink a least eight glasses a day you would see a huge improvement in your skin".** *NO amount of oil of Olay will moisture your skin as water and nourishing food which may prove to be a better investment in having and maintaining lustrous skin and glowing health.*

Truth is we are water beings from the sperm seaman/semen to the egg we function in water.

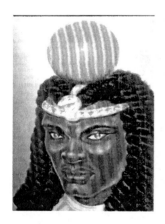

RE re

The word Re re or tone Ray in TAMARE is the final principle in our school. This tone brings together all other tones and is a key element in all things.

For example:
Music: Do Ray Mi So La (solar) Te Do
Science: Resonance, Regeneration, Relativity, Resolution, Response, Respiration
Art: Re-creation
Mathematics: Reciprocal, Reflection, Reflex, Rectangle and Revolution.

Re align Re member Re spect Re turn this is an oscillation a vibratory rate of creation bringing something anything into existence and this creation is constant like thoughts. Re is to do again and again and again. That is why it is a prefix word and sound in every repeated action in the Dictionary (definitionary), and if any form of creation is hidden it will eventually be exposed, again and again by the physical or spiritual sun. This being is one we must acquaint ourselves with as this is The Most High being. Supreme Being of supreme beings Ra has the Greeks had many of us using is the later form of Re (Ray) of ancient Egypt. Re was the name given to the sun by the Egyptians. RE is the sun or Solar deity, the fire principle dealing with heat, light, vitality and knowledge.

The physical sun of our solar system is symbolic as it is the first born giving birth to our planets and is so vital to our lives if the sun was blocked out for an entire day everything on this planet will begin to die.

The sun is about 93 million miles away its temperature on the surface is around 9,980F and at its core the temperature is approx 27,000,0000F this is to say that the Ancient Afrikans are spot on when they relate themselves and all things in creation to the number 9. RE origins was in the water of Nun having his eyes and mouth shut. After becoming tired of his inactivity he climbed from the darkness showing himself in all his glory. RE predates Allah who's plural is Allahumma (Quran 5 times 3:26, 3:17, 8:32, 10:10, 39:36) The word means "Oh Allah the source" Allahumma is another word that was derived from the Hebrew word Eloheem found in the Torah 430 times, meaning *"These beings* "or "*A group of Elohs, the Gods"*. The attributes of Allah coincide with the 99 elements which can be traced further back to the 99 Ancient ancestors or Neters which I will show further in this book. The 36th Attribute of Allah called Al Aliyu "The Most High" is also the name of the 86th chapter of the Koran today which was originally 86th chapter called Suwrah Al Ala "Chapter of The Most High". The 36th attribute of Allah Al Aliyu "The Most High" muslims use when they say "Allahu Subhanna Wa Ta' Ala- Glory be to Allah The Most High", or in shorten "Allah Ta'Ala – Allah The Most High" As in Genesis 14:18 and Koran 87:1 "The Most High God" which in Hebrew is Elyuwn Elyuwn El it can be found in the bible a total of 43 times.

The 93rd Attribute of Allah is "Al Nuwr –The Light", Koran 24:35 'The source, Allah is the Nuwr 'light of the samawati, skies and the planet earth, RE the visible emblem of the most high Anu and was regarded as the head of the YAHWEH meaning "He who is, who he is" or the NETERU, NETERS, Nature, the personification of the 99 elements, the Elders, Ancestors. Re has many forms. One that was most important was the one where he is seen with a falcon head wearing a solar disk and ureas.

PA RE the sun is the source of life and without this source I repeat all on this planet will die as the ecosystems of earth is sustained by Re. Our ancients recognised this crucial source, and were seen to be sun worshippers. This is but a misinterpretation on the part of those who robbed the graves, tombs and temples of ancient Khemet. The actual source of sun worship was originally the sun inside, not the sun outside but as in reference to the solar plexus our central system and second brain also known as central intelligence. As was taught by The Supreme Spiritual Master Amunnubi RoakhPtah, that *"Re symbolises Universal Consciousness, and in man individual consciousness. Consciousness is the receiving capacity of the soul or individual intelligence"*.

The Solar plexus sits within the centre of our digestive system the carrier of our emotions. The digestion begins at the mouth and ends at the rectum. The Solar plexus is also depicted with the colour yellow which is the colour of intellect. We are sun/solar beings Ether-utopians, Ethiopians born and descended from RE

RE is attributed as the all seeing eye of which all the occultist are aware of yet by many has been taught as the evil eye which is misinformation in order to sodden the name of our ancestor and also for the superstitious ones to be controlled by fear altering the steps to the facts about the truth behind our bondage who we are where we came from and of course where we are going. This all Seeing Eye comes from the ability to be present and consciously aware. To be present and not seen is the skill of invisibility, which leads to **Amun.** Amun is the hidden principle of Re and Re is the personification of Amun. Amun, who is also called Amen, Amin, Ameen Iman, Imani and Mu'min; is still being worshipped today by Jews, Christians and Muslims; all their prayers end with Amen meaning *'faith'.*

These principles are the foundation and make up of you the Smai *Afrikan Yogi* who prescribes to Wu- Nuwaupu the worker of *'nine mind'.*

The Mutalub/student of smai is well aware of these principles; they are well aware of the deities/guardians that govern them and strive to grasp the inner workings of the cosmology pertaining to his/herself, also known as the inner mysteries as well as the outer mysteries. This is the very thing that they teach.

This is the essential behind the symbology. They progress further as they are now rooted into the Nine. The smai practitioner utilises the 'Science of Nine Ether'; which in essence is a series of principles. It is evident that these principles have to some become more of a religion. Religions breeds hatred, separation, racism, ignorance and war as the ego is an entity that feels disconnected from All. The ego perceives itself constantly under threat and seeks out constant conflict within and without. Within religions the personalities (Jesus Buddha Muhammad Moses) take over the teachings giving birth to further personalities (Pastors Missionaries Monks Rabbis and Imams) staunch followers and egotistic entities who strip the higher teachings down into a series of dos and don'ts, good and bad a series of polarities and dichotomies.

These parameters as human beings we struggle with and will constantly struggle with for these lower mysteries do not allow for GOD consciousness to truly prevail as they do not enhance our divinity they eventually becomes a matrix. Like all religions when stripped down to its bare essential the underlining principles lead one to a higher state of consciousness. Wu-Nuwaupu (God Consciousness) can in no way be mentally understood and there is no intellectual agreement. Wu-Nuwaupu (God Consciousness) must be felt completely with every cell of your body and every connection of your being Wu-Nuwaupu (God Consciousness) is unspoken, unwritten, the un-manifested. The time is truly now when you The Afrikan must realise that science you prescribe to cannot be found outside of yourself in any church, synogogue, temple, tabernacle or alter it can only be found waiting in silence within where the truth of you, your wants your wishes and the universe move as one flow, like a stream of universal beauty. There is your power and your connection with your divine self. The practice of Afrikan Yoga 'smai' is key component in my realisation of this fact as I used movement, body awareness, breath and meditation (inner stillness) to facilitate a higher consciousness; a journey where emotions and ego are watched all the way. This is journey where intensity, presence and living are evenly matched in a pool of timelessness, no-thing and no separation.

This journey we really call transformation as the ancient alchemist spoke of from base metals into gold. Where you shine like the sun and no negativity can reside in you and no negativity can sit beside you and not be transformed.

"I am the Great One, the son of a Great One. I am the Fiery One, the son of a Fiery One, whose head was restored to him after it had been cut off. The head of Osiris, the Risen Saviour, is not taken from him and my head shall not be taken from me. I have risen up and knitted myself together. I have made myself whole. I renew myself and grow young again. I am one with Osiris, Lord of Eternity".

The book Coming Forth by Day, **Atum**

The Radience of a Great Master Teacher's Tool

"The greatest challenge for the initiate is to refrain from taking sides in the seeming conflicts of life. All adversities exist for the sake of making demands upon the individual to reach into the depths of his/her spirit to awaken the spiritual power to overcome them. One cannot push exert force if there is no opposition, there can be no manifestation of spiritual power without adversity. All is peace. Hetep.

Ra Un Nefer Amen, Medu Neter Vol 1.

I know this to be true seeing the countless obstacles in life I have personally encountered as a means to my growth and seeing the conflicts many family and friends have suffered to a bitter end or to overwhelming joy and expansion of their lives. The master tool in the recognitions of such onslaughts on ones hetep/peace is the wisdom of Tehuti an invaluable resource of understanding the laws of mind. However, these laws are themselves illusions, a matrix of which we must rise above or delve deeper in being order to be one, to reconnect to our true self the self connected to all things. They must be overstood.

Before speaking about TEHUTI and the principles also known as laws, let me relay an experience that gave me a deeper insight to this master.

While practising Vipassana Meditation under the guidance of S.N Goenka a teacher of Indian descent born in Burma and devout Buddhist also a teacher of thousands of people in more than 350 courses in India and other countries, East and West who had become a master of Meditation I received what is known as internal insight. The technique which S.N Goenka teaches represents a tradition that is traced back to the Buddha. In short the technique is one of self-observation that shows reality in its two aspects, inner and outer. In the language of India at the time of Buddha, *passana* meant to look, to see things in the ordinary way; but *vipassana* is to observe things as they really are, not just as they seem to be. Apparent truth had to be penetrated, until one reaches the ultimate truth of the entire mental and physical structure.

During this time a question kept on rearing its head. Who is Buddha?

Strict observations of silence called Noble Silence for 9 days and 10 hrs of meditation a day had to be adhered to for 10 days (courses can last up to 30

54

days). In the first two days when permitted I began to ask the assistant teachers about Buddha, Of course short and brief answers where returned. Guatama Buddah was not the first; there where many Buddhas, and Guatema was part of a spiritual linage. Listening to the discourses of S.N Goenka, the axioms he used from the teachings of Buddha resembled the **Hah Kha**, the sacred wisdom teachings of Tehuti, also known as the greater mysteries which gave birth to the lesser mysteries: Christianity, Judaism and Islam. I found myself in the wisdom school, the school of Tehuti *naturally*. The **Hah kha** resurfaced today by the Spiritual Master teacher, Amon Nubi Roakhptah. I was able to recognise all the axioms presented and this intensified my question. So who was the first Buddha? In exploring my structure day after day during meditation the answer sparked that this Buddha who gave birth to a line of spiritual aspirants is no other than The Grand Heirophant Tehuti himself. Guatema Buddha was a student of Dravidian yogi's as well as Tehuti. Guatema proved the maxims of the original teachings for himself by sitting for long periods of time in meditation. "Be still and know that I Am God". This speaks of the God within, the divine self and instructs an awakening to pure consciousness devoid of attachments and the ramblings of the mind. Tehuti or in Greek Thoth where we get the word 'thought' derived certain principles, maxims and axioms to assist the realising of true consciousness. Buddha means the awakened one. This literally means that you can be Buddha as and when you awaken in your own lifetime, today and not some distant future, and not just and exclusive experience of Siddartha Guatema has the Buddhist believe.

Note: I recommend that all smai/yoga aspirants take up this practise and to perform 9 days of Noble silence with 10 full hours of Meditation daily, once a year to maintain and develop their inner wisdom. I'll explain my reasoning behind this by adding the comments of Dr Muata Ashby from his book African Origins of Civilization, Religion and Yoga Spirituality.

"The origins of Hatha Yoga were clearly in Buddhism and not in Hinduism since we find evidence of rejection of Hatha Yoga by the Hindu sages. Hatha Yoga is clearly rejected in the Laghu-Yoga –Vaisistha (5.6.86, 92), which maintains that it merely leads to pain; some of critisms, especially against the magical undercurrents". Dr Muata Ashby continues further saying *"Specifically, Tantric Buddhism gave rise to the earliest practice of certain postures as a means to enhance spiritual evolution. Before this time, the only reference to asana or posture was the sitting posture for meditation mentioned in the Raja Yoga Sutras by Pantanjali. STHIRA SUKHAM ASANAM STHIRA: Steady. SUKHAM: Comfortable. ASANAM: Pose (for meditation) meaning: A seated pose (for meditation) that is steady and comfortable is called Asana*

To attain success in the practice of concentration, meditation and Samadhi, an aspirant begins by developing steadiness of a meditative pose.

Buddhist records show that early Buddhist had visited Memphis (Sakkara/Tattu the nome or city of Ptah, author's addition) and set up a settlement there. Henceforth Buddhism begins to develop similar iconographies including the Divinity sitting on the lotus, similar to those of ancient Egypt.

To encase this further "In ancient Kamit there were at least 24 postures in the spiritual practice prior to the time of Pantajali. In the practice of Kamitian Tjef Neteru (Egyptian Hatha Yoga) the "magic" consist in using postures to engender certain alignments with spiritual energies and cosmic forces. This is the kind of practice repudiated by the Hindu sages and adopted by the Tantric Buddhists. Between the years 100 A.C.E. and 1000 A.C.E. the Buddhist Kaula school developed some postures. Then Goraksha developed what is regarded by present day Hatha Yoga practicioners as a practice similar to the present day. However, the number postures only reached 15 at the time of Hatha Yoga Pradipika scripture. The Mysore family was instrumental in the development since they were strong patrons of Hatha Yoga. Subsequent teachers developed more postures and vinyasa (sequences of poses synchronised with the breath) [which was not practised in early Indian Hatha Yoga] up to the 20th century where there are over 200. The teacher Krishnamacharya said he had learned from a yoga teacher in Tibet. Krishnamacharya's first writings, which cited the Stitattvandihi as a source, also featured vinyasa that Krishnamacharya said he had learned form a teacher in Tibet. So the practise of the postures in India does not extend to ancient times and did not begin in India with Hinduism but with Buddhism and Buddhism was associated with the Ancient Egyptian city of Memphis where postures and spiritual magic were practised previously".

The father of "magic" is Tehuti and in order to perform magic and not tricks there is great emphasis on mastering your thoughts and controlling your mind which can only be achieved through meditation. The Greeks had translated the name Tehuti to Thoth, which when observed seems innocent and just a transliteration. However, Thoth gives us the word thought, and it is thoughts that causes us to miss constantly the ultimate reality, pure joy, pure love and freedom found in the state of 'NOW' only to osscilate between the past and future, good and bad meaning being in a state of duality. That is why as descendents of these great masters and ancestors we can not afford to lean too much on Greek translations of our ancient names and places. Return to the Great Master's tool meditation and regain the mastery of your mind within this process you have access to all the answers you need.

Buddha was Black, that's why his woolly hair is always shown in small tight curls, pepper corn style or corn rows. Early sculptures of him clearly reveal his Aficoid features… wide nose and full lips. So was Zaha of Japan, Fu-Hsi of China, Tyr of Scandinavia, Quetzalcoatl of Mexico, Sommonacom of Siam and Isis of Egypt and Rome. Krishna of India was "blue-black".

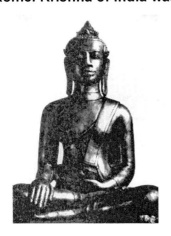

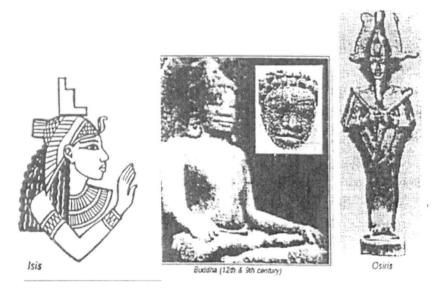

Isis

Buddha (12th & 9th century)

Osiris

These great sages cannot be denied and to say they were otherwise when drawn images and carved stone depicts them Afrikan is to reveal a mental health and pathological issue.

Tehuti/Djehuti tehuti

Named by the Greeks (the so called foundation of European thought and culture) Thoth had many names: Tehuty, dihuty, Dhouti, Thout, Zehuti, Sheps, Lord of the Khemenu. Father time

Djehuty "Leader" Ibis-headed Lord of Time, Writing and Wisdom, Djehuty is a scribe who wrote the story of our reality.

The name Thoth means 'Truth' and 'Time'. Thoth was the Master architect who created the blueprint of our reality based on the mathematics of sacred geometry and placed it in Grids (A Matrix) for us to experience and learn.

It also has been said that he invented the hieroglyphic script and negotiated five extra days from the moon in order to perfect the 365-day year. As a result of these mythological connections, he is also known as the diety of the moon.and the moon cycle. Djehuty is the patron of writers, teachers, accountants and all persons involved in the dissemination of knowledge, writing and/or calculation. His consorts are alternately **Ma'at**, Netert of Truth and Order; or Seshat, patroness of recordkeeping, libraries and the foundation of buildings.

It was Tehuti who helped Aset work the ritual to bring Asaru back from the dead, and who drove the magical poison of Set from her son, Haru with the power of his magic. He was Haru's supporter during the young deity deadly battle with his uncle Set, helping Haru with his wisdom and magic. It was Tehuti who brought Tefnut, who left Egypt for Nubia in a sulk after an argument with her father, back to heaven to be re-united with Re (Sun). When Re retired from the Earth, (the end of the sun cycle) he appointed Tehuti and told him of his desire to create a Light-soul in the Duat and in the Land of the Caves, and it was over this region that the sun god appointed Tehuti to rule, (moon cycle) ordering him to keep a register of those who were there, and to mete out just punishments to them. Tehuti became the representation of Re in the afterlife, seen at the judgment of the dead in the 'Halls of the Double Ma'at'.

You see the sun-cycle and moon cycle are actually equinoxes of the universe Tehuti was the 'god of the equilibrium' and considered depictions of him as the 'Master of the Balance' to indicate that he was associated with the equinoxes the time when the day and the night were evenly balanced.

Djehuty is the nominal head of the Ogdoad (group of eight Names of Netjer) honored at the city of Khemenu (Hermopolis of the Greeks), overseeing four pairs of natural synergies: Eternity (Heh/Hehet), Darkness (Kek/Keket), Water/Potentiality (Nun/Nunet) and Wind/Invisibility (Amen/Amenet).

The 9 principles of Tehuti Related to Yoga

The 9 principles of Tehuti where replace by what is now known as the Seven Hermetic Laws below are the 9 principles also known as doctrines.

1. Mental (please refer to Meditation exercises).

We must not confuse mental with mind and mind with general brain function one sole purpose is to interpret impulses to give and receive information from the various nerves in and on the physical body. Mental or consciousness is beyond mind. That only is to say that the mind does not merely exist in ones skull but is a pervasive entity of the human being as explained in the 9 principles.

"All is mental and each has a mind" Tehuti

"Each individual has a mind and is fed by the same mental reservoir, which enables each individual to grasp the laws of the mental, and to apply the same to his/her well being and advancement. That's being in touch with the real god.

   With the **ANKH** "Master-Key" in his/her possession the student may unlock the many doors of the mental and psychic temple of Right Knowledge, Right Wisdom and Right Overstanding, and enter the same freely using the God mind you have or the mind of mental which is God. This explains the true nature of energy, power and matter, existence and why and how all these are subordinate to the mastery of the mind. This clarifys that each mind is a slave to mental, the force of ether, which controls the action of matter".

Dr Malachi Z York, The Sacred Wisdom

The mental is an area that feeds the mind. The purpose of Afrikan Yoga is to tame the mind and release it's potency through the realisation and reconnection of the mental reservoir through meditation (stillness) and postures (movement).
Gushing forth clarity with this realisation the practitioner can gain control of their destiny by utilising the principle of mental. What ever happens to me or does not happen to me is within mind. One is capable of healing themselves as they now know that sickness and instability arises from the unconscious mind where there may be a feeling of disconnection with one self; the 'Self/Being', which is seated

in supreme consciousness. Dr Malachi AmunNebu RE Akh Tah mentions the 'force of ether'. This force is inter-layered with our over-soul with is the Akh (Etheric) you or "Etheric Body" which is also known as the 'spiritual plane; over lapping 'the plane of force'. This is channelled through the Mer seat or third eye Arush (Chakra). The plane of material existence is subjected to the plane of force in the same way one is able with the use of the mind (re-member; now the mind that is aware of the interconnectivity of all things and knows it is within **"Pa Tempta"** *"The All"*) to magnetise your wants and wishes, however, be careful what you wish for and use 'Right Wisdom'.

2. Correspondence

"As above, so below; as below, so above" — *The Kybalion*

This Principle embodies the truth that there is always a Correspondence between the laws and phenomena of the various planes of Being and Life. The old Hermetic axiom ran in these words: "*As above, so below; as below, so above*".

"*In these words 'as above so below'; will mislead you into thinking that there are two directions, when infact there is no directions at all. Even your own planet is going nowhere, around and back again. So time is going nowhere. And the grasping of this doctrine gives one the means of solving many a blinding paradox and hidden secret of Nature at work in all things.*

Dr Malachi Z York, The Sacred Wisdom

There are planes beyond our knowing: but when we apply the Principle of Correspondence to them, we are able to understand much that would otherwise be unknowable to us. This Principle is of universal application and manifestation on the various planes of the material, mental, and spiritual universe — it is a Universal Law. The ancient Smai considered this Principle to be one of the most important mental instruments by which man was able to pry aside the obstacles, which hid the 'Unknown' from view. To ask a question and to be able to see and recognise the answer is due to the realisation that all corresponds, interconnected and has a relationship. With patience and the application of observation answers are easier to come by. Afrikan Yoga utilises the principle in relation to body, mind and spirit when one is able to form a sanuy/posture and be aware of the corresponding relationship and effect of the corresponding organ, gland, mental stimuli and spiritual resonance created by the form in line with breath. The Ancient smai practitioner led the way and mapped out various movements and sounds to which has their correspondence with internal organs through to the planets in our solar system. I give thanks for their wisdom and tireless efforts of self-mastery in order to achieve this and to leave with us a legacy in the movements of Pa Neteru Tamare Smai Afrikan Yoga.

3. Vibration

"Nothing rests; everything moves; everything vibrates" — The Kybalion

This principle embodies the truth that "everything is in motion"; "everything vibrates"; "Nothing is at rest"; — facts which Modern Science endorses and which each new scientific discovery tends to verify. And yet this Hermetic Principle was enunciated thousands of years ago by the Masters of Ancient Egypt.

This Principle explains that the differences between different manifestations of Matter, Energy, Mind, and even Spirit, result largely from varying rates of Vibration. From THE ALL, which is Pure Spirit, down to the grossest form of Matter, all is in vibration: the higher the vibration, the higher the position in the scale. The vibration of Spirit is at such an infinite rate of intensity and rapidity that it is practically at rest — just as a rapidly moving wheel seems to be motionless. And at the other end of the scale, there are gross forms of matter whose vibrations are so low as to seem at rest. Between these poles, there are millions upon millions of varying degrees of vibration. From corpuscle and electron, atom and molecule, to worlds and galaxies, everything is in vibratory motion. This is also true on the planes of energy and force (which are but varying degrees of vibration); and also on the mental planes (whose states depend upon vibrations); and even on the spiritual planes. An understanding of this Principle, with the appropriate formulas, enables Tamare Smai students to control their own mental vibrations as well as those of others. The Masters also apply this Principle to the conquering of Natural phenomena in various ways. One of the old writers says: "*He who understands the Principle of Vibration has grasped the 'SEKHEM' sceptre of power*". With the right vibrational charge one is able to accomplish anything. To reiterate this law is the basis for particle physics. It is within this law that resonance is applied to change matter by changing energy. We change things by applying the right frequency or intensity to a subject, object. This is why in Afrikan Yoga we use tones in our movements and also why we Gaanum/Hika Chant as we are summoning light into the body like an invisible laser to heal the corresponding organs. This is also applied to affirmations, as they are commands and decrees consisting of word-sound, tone, visualisation and intensity all equalling vibrations of will. We are creators of our reality through the vibrations that resonates from our thoughts into the universe.

4. Polarity

The Great Master taught…
"Everything is dual; everything has poles; everything has its pair of opposites; likes and unlike are the same; opposites are identical in nature; but different in degree; extremes meet; all truths are but half-truths; all paradoxes may be reconciled". This doctrine has to be understood in order to bring balance to your being, we are often instructed by master sages to be wary of extremes. Overstand that extreme ends or poles are one and the same, hot and cold which are polarities of degrees of heat. This is to say can you find where hot ends and cold begins. Try this stand in a room with a fire or heater and a door exiting to outside and walk to one end of the room to the other just to see where hot and cold begins. This will demonstrate the meaning of duality being the same. It really is down to where you are at mentally. Hard and soft, big and small, positive and negative, like and dislike and at times we experience love and hate all are oscillating vibrations or degrees of mental will, this the Smai student and mystic uses to transmute evil into good, a worthless thing into something of use. Remember mutalub your perception of the world is a reflection of your state of consciousness. The mastery of the principle of polarity or what is known as "The Art of Polarisation" or "Mental Alchemy" was and is practised by the students of Tehuti. Smai practitioners who devote themselves to this 'Art' will be able to perform transformation of polarity within them selves at will and therefore change the polarity of others. As was taught by AmunnubiRuachPtah turn "evil in to good" In relation to Smai *hanua*at movements or *ragulaat* exercises the smai student avoid extremes so the stretch should always be in the bounds of comfortability and devoid of competition with class members or with self (Ego). The stretch with the use of "Mental Alchemy" will transmute your feelings towards a movement or sanuy/posture creating positivity where there once was a negative attitude therefore creating a barrier to achieving the movement.

5. Rhythm (please refer to Hudu/Movement)

The Great Master taught…
Everything flows out and in, everything has its tides, all things rise and fall, the pendulum swing manifest in everything, the measure of the swing to the right is the measure of the swing to the left, rhythm compensates. To swing to and fro you need a point of origin and a fixed spot, as to where the cord hangs from, and

the first movement to start the swing. Yet all of this is in The All. This is a physical principle. A motive principle.

This principle of rhythm recognises the sacred truth of universal law of the passing away and the coming to be of the circular flow of things. "What goes around comes around" (but not always the same way). That "trouble does not last always" [and that] "joy can be found in the morning". These old African phrases are an embodiment of rhythm illustrated by the pendulum swing.

In Tamare Smai African Yoga this principle has to be understood by the student/practitioner has the aim is to attain self mastery and be the holder of the pendulum where you control the rate, speed and eventually suspend swinging to a level of balance between polarities. This at times is unconsciously done however; when consciously done that's when the master in you appears.

On a physical level as well as the principle many Afrikans now living in the West suffer from 'Rhythm Dis-ease'. Many are no longer in tune with their bodies and the subtleties of their soul. So are unable to dance the womb dance or the movements of Pa Netert Tefnut and Het-Heru. As can be seen in various Carnival or 'Bashment' dance hall and African dances today.

I have witnessed the embarrassment first hand when a sister or brother cannot flow rhythmically with the elements around them. Jarred by computer screens, western clothing, 9-5 stress laden city living lifestyles, now copying dances that only mimic movements inspired by joyous living in the sun. The movements become vague and almost unrecognisable to the traditional durational movements of adoration coming from Nomes and villages throughout Afrika.

They are remnants of powerful healing tools of the spirit, mind and body.

Afrikan Yoga removes your stiffness and releases energy flow through out the body to such an extent that you are able to be aware of your flexibility and your potential to be fully mobile. Reclaim your rhythm and dance more in adoration and gratitude of your life, your ancestors and your divinity.

6. Cause and Effect

"Every Cause has its Effect; every Effect has its Cause; everything happens according to Law; Chance is but a name for Law not recognised; there are many planes of causation, but nothing escapes the Law". — The Kybalion

"Nothing manifest in the effect, unless it is in the cause"

Amon Nubi Roakh Ptah

The doctrine of cause and effect is that nothing is left to chance, chance and luck are illusions and all things are interrelated by a cause that will manifest an effect that becomes another cause. There are vary degrees of this law in all dimensions and nothing escapes the law, as a student who may well be a master if you overstand this law. For most are subject to cause unaware of it and it's effect so are controlled, manipulated and pawned in 'the game of life' however, you may use this law to become movers and even rulers in the game of life where you move and make things happen by will. It is said nothing escapes this law has you are still subject to obey the law on higher planes of existence, however, you may become masters, rulers, movers and shakers on your plane of existence. This principle applied to Smai is the understanding of movement and breath it's cause is the desire, the will and the posture and its effects the mental, physiological and spiritual benefits etc. Study each sanuy/posture within this book to find the effects of them in order to master imbalances in the KHAT (body) KA (spirit) BA (soul) KHU (mental) you.

7. Gender (please refer to Taful Sanuy)

The Great Master taught…
The doctrine of Gender works ever in the direction of generation, regeneration and creation. Everything and every person contains the two elements or doctrines within it him or her. Every male thing has the female element also; every female contains the male doctrine.

It has been said *'that spirit has no gender'*. So when you move beyond physical forms and physical thought processes, gender is non existent has your polarities are viewed as one. In the womb genderisation is formed in the second trimester and is appeared where one also forms their spiritual and mental interactions (ref Afrikan Holistic Health by Dr Llaila O Afrika) This is to say during your creation of physical person(s) in this period as a foetus your sex, mental and spiritual preferences also is formed and this is heavily influenced by your parents interactions, state of mind, nutritional intake and times of solar and lunar positioning. In the west there is some what of a confusion where gender swapping is actively encouraged with very little understanding of 'Gender Principles' the result is mental and physical violence on the populace by the populace, we unconsciously and consciously hurt each other in this state of ignorance.

Male and female principles are our means of communication, creativity and harmonising all aspects of our existence on this plane. All physical beings, objects and even laws are goverened by the principle of gender.

In our cosmology our explanation of the sciences called mysteries we communicate via

TA MU NEFU SET [Earth Water Air Fire], which is the feminine principle. **1. Think 2. Feel (Receive) 3. Process 4. Act**.

TA NEFU MU SET [Earth Air Water Fire] is the Male principle. **1.Think 2. Process 3. Feel (Receive) 4. Act**.

Its important to note when in engaging in movement and stillness you are having a relationship with these principle within and without your person and to overstand them is to know when they are in effect in your being and to know what being is communicating with you. When communicating into the feminine energy as a male you will switch to TA MU NEFU SET, which is [Think Feel/Receive/Process Act]

Communication with the male energy you switch to TA NEFU MU SET [Think Process Feel/Receive Act]. Now men take note a man thinks first then feels and a woman feels first then process. When speaking with a woman you better tell her how you feel first. The same concern for the ladies you better tell the brother what you think prior to how you feel. This will avoid many unwanted arguments (However, some arguments are not to be avoided as they assist your understanding and growth as long as you are observing your feelings and self you can tell what principle you are speaking in and where the person you are conversing with is coming from). Disharmony can be caused when one is unaware or ignores the facts of this great principle. The Mutalub/Student is free to express the masculine and feminine principles in the form of 'Shen' and 'Sham', hard and soft, inverted and extroverted applied in AfrikanYoga as the Gender principles relate to the Sanuyaat forms. While at the same time they are fused in the one being as there is no gender. This is reiterated in the doctrines of Tehuti.

"Gender is in everything; everything has its masculine and feminine principles; gender manifests on all planes. Again there is no real gender except what appears in the physical realm and in the spiritual realm. You are not male or female, you are god".

The Sacred Wisdom

8. Growth

The doctrine of growth encompasses all principles of creation. The doctrine of growth and creation has been primarily left out of the 7 hermetic laws. Ammonubi Roachptah teaches that this principle must make you Pa mutalub/the student realise that all things that exist on the physical plane grew he uses the term created and this creation created itself out of pre-existing matter or energy also known as dark-matter. Even your god concept grew out of darkness and god is not separated from creation but apart.

'The root reality of creation is that the very word means to grow. As habits grow, thoughts grow, knowledge grows, illness grows, bacteria grows, the mind grows but through information channelled from an etheric cord the mental, the reservoir of outtellect, and the source from which the mind is fed intellect. These are realities, substantial realities, material realities. The universe is a pheneomenon of life that grew into existence'.

This relates has we see ourselves grow materially and mentally it also has to be recognised that growth in part can be stubbed however, something is always growing and it is for the student to be aware of this growth.

Enlightened travellers take care to leave everything beautifully.
Enlightened speakers take care to explore and explain every leaf.
Enlightened science is self evident; enlightened discussion self fulfilling.
Enlightened holism generates free energy.
Enlightened beings have time for everyone and ignore noone.
They pay attention to every last thing, ignoring nothing.
So they are called enlightened.
Just as the enlightened offer examples to the confounded and the confuse,
so do the confounded offer opportunities for the enlightened to shine.
To avoid appreciating exemplary beings, or to avoid the opportunity of shining,
would be a mistake whoever you are.
Realising this subtle interplay is vital to the learning and burgeoning of right relationships; thus vital to evolution.

27 Tao Teh Ching by Lao Tzu

9. Breath

The Smai mutalub/student practices exercises by which they attains control of

67

their body, and is enabled to send to any organ or part an increased flow of Sekhem vital force, thereby strengthening and invigorating the part or organ. He/she knows all that his Western scientific brother knows about the physiological effect of correct breathing, but he/she also knows that the air contains more than oxygen and hydrogen and nitrogen, and that something more is accomplished than the mere oxygenating of the blood.

He/She knows something about Sekhem of which his/her Western counterpart is ignorant, and he is fully aware of the nature and manner of handling that great principle of energy, and is fully informed as to its effect upon the human body and mind. He knows that by rhythmical breathing one may bring himself into harmonious vibration with nature, and aid in the unfoldment of his latent powers. He knows that by controlled breathing he may not only cure disease in himself and others, but also practically do away with fear and worry and the baser emotions

(Hatha Yoga by Yogi Ramacharaka)

The Smai Complete Breath

The Smai Complete Breath is the fundamental breath of the entire Smai Science of Breath, and the student must fully acquaint himself with it, and master it perfectly before he can hope to obtain results from the other forms of breath mentioned and given in this book. He should not be content with half-learning it, but should go to work in earnest until it becomes his natural method of breathing. This will require work, time and patience, but without these things nothing is ever accomplished. There is no shortcut to the Science of Breath, and the student must be prepared to practice and study in earnest if he expects to receive results. The results obtained by a complete mastery of the Science of Breath are great, and no one who has attained them would willingly go back to the old methods, and he will tell his friends that he considers himself amply repaid for all his work. I say these things now, that you may fully understand the necessity and importance of mastering this fundamental method of Yogi Breathing, instead of passing it by and trying some of the attractive looking variations given later on in this book. Again, we say to you: Start right, and right results will follow; but neglect your foundations and your entire building will topple over sooner or later. Perhaps the better way to teach you how to develop the Smai Complete Breath, would be to give you simple directions regarding the breath itself, and then follow up the same with general remarks concerning it, and then later on giving exercises for developing the chest, muscles and lungs which have been allowed to remain in an undeveloped condition by imperfect methods of breathing. Right here we wish to say that this Complete Breath is not a forced or abnormal thing, but on the contrary it is a going back to first principles-a return to Nature. The healthy adult savage and the healthy infant of civilization both breathe in this manner, but civilized man has adopted unnatural methods of living, clothing, etc., and has lost his birthright. And we wish to remind the reader that the Complete Breath does not necessarily call for the complete filling of the lungs at every inhalation. One may inhale the average amount of air, using the Complete Breathing Method and distributing the air inhaled, be the quantity large or small, to all parts of the lungs. But one should inhale a series of full Complete Breaths several times a day, whenever opportunity offers, in order to keep the system in good order and condition.

The following simple exercise will give you a clear idea of what the Complete Breath is:

(1) Stand or sit erect. Breathing through the nostrils, inhale steadily, first filling the lower part of the lungs, which is accomplished by bringing into play the diaphragm, which descending exerts a gentle pressure on the abdominal organs, pushing forward the front walls of the abdomen. Then fill the middle part of the lungs, pushing out the lower ribs, breastbone and chest. Then fill the higher portion of the lungs, protruding the upper chest, thus lifting the chest, including the upper six or sever pairs of ribs. In the final movement, the lower part of the abdomen will be slightly drawn in, which movement gives the lungs a support and also helps to fill the highest part of the lungs. At first reading it may appear that this breath consists of three distinct movements. This, however, is not the correct idea. The inhalation is continuous, the entire chest cavity from the lowered diaphragm to the highest point of the chest in the region of the collarbone, being expanded with a uniform movement. Avoid a jerky series of inhalations, and strive to attain a steady continuous action. Practice will soon overcome the tendency to divide the inhalation into three movements, and will result in a uniform continuous breath. You will be able to complete the inhalation in a couple of seconds after a little practice.

(2) Retain the breath a few seconds.

(3) Exhale quite slowly, holding the chest in a firm position, and drawing the abdomen in a little and lifting it upward slowly as the air leaves the lungs. When the air is entirely exhaled, relax the chest and abdomen. A little practice will render this part of the exercise easy, and the movement once acquired will be afterwards performed almost automatically. It will be seen that by this method of breathing all parts of the respiratory apparatus is brought into action, and all parts of the lungs, including the most remote air cells, are exercised. The chest cavity is expanded in all directions. You

will also notice that the Complete Breath is really a combination of Low, Mid and High Breaths, succeeding each other rapidly in the order given, in such a manner as to form one uniform, continuous, complete breath.

You will find it quite a help to you if you will practice this breath before a large mirror, placing the hands lightly over the abdomen so that you may feel the movements. At the end of the inhalation, it is well to occasionally slightly elevate the shoulders, thus raising the collarbone and allowing the air to pass freely into the small upper lobe of the right lung, which place is sometimes the breeding place of tuberculosis.

At the beginning of practice, you may have more or less trouble in acquiring the Complete Breath, but a little practice will make perfect, and when you have once acquired it you will never willingly return to the old methods.

In imperfect or shallow breathing, only a portion of the lung cells are brought into play, and a great portion of the lung capacity is lost, the system suffering in proportion to the amount of under-oxygenation. The lower animals, in their native state, breathe naturally, and primitive man undoubtedly did the same. The abnormal manner of living adopted by so called civilized man which really means western man - the shadow that follows upon civilization - has robbed us of our awareness of breathing and our natural habits of breathing, and human beings has greatly suffered thereby. Our only physical salvation is to "get back to Nature". To be grounded and connected with mother/father earth.

Grounding is being present in the here and now, connected to earth and all things. However, sitting in easy pose or Nefertem posture is grounding.

Meditation is the ultimate grounding tool. 10 min of silence and stillness a day and build up to 1hour.

When Breathing what should I do/visualise/be?

Try your Rhythmic breathing to 4. If one counts to 4 for inhalation one must use the same for exhalation if you count to 4 then your rest or relaxation will be 2 counts also your retention 2 counts so that you maintain a 2:1 ratio between inhalation and retention and exhalation and relaxation. You can build this up to 8 counts when you have perfected and comfortable with 4 counts

There are many things one can visualise during Smai breathing. Self-Healing ailments and areas of the body including the 'oversoul', concentrating on desired outcomes etc. However, for now during Smai breathing one should keep the mouth closed, use the imagination (the will and visualisation) to control the passage of air entering the body. Visualise the breath entering the nasal passages and floating to the back of the throat and down into your being and visualise the expulsion of air back up and out through the nasal passages.

What should you be? Well be relaxed and either lie down or stand or sit in a comfortable position with your spine straight and your head erect (just as we do in class). The standing position is considered to be the ideal position for a number of breathing techniques due to the fact that the distribution of muscular stress is fairly even throughout the entire body especially if the head is erect, the back is kept straight, the feet is slightly apart and the arms are hanged loosely by the sides. However, you can still do this on the bus or at home.

The breathing technique that improves the co-ordination of several systems of the body is both the Smai Complete Union Breathing technique, which incorporates all three clavicles, intercostals and diaphragm breathing "Fug shallow/Bayna mid breathing and Tat low/diaphragm". This is where the expansion of the diaphragm, ribs, sternum and lungs come into play by steady slow and continuous inhalation of air through the nose and an equal exhalation occurs to expel the air keeping the mouth closed.

The Rhythmic breathing technique, is used where again practise is slow and deliberate/conscious or what can be called intelligent breathing where the student controls the time for inhalation retention, exhalation and rest/relaxation repeating the cycle. Both the circulatory and respiratory system rhythmic co-ordination benefits significantly as well as other systems of the body.

Sekhem... Spark of Life

SEKHEM is **SE**- The creative principle, the source of spirit and life force
SE- The human soul.
KHEM - Black not in terms of colour, tone or mood but as supreme balance the true meaning of black, when viewing this meaning in metaphysics and science we have to look at melanin and carbon. Melanin is a conductor and battery and carbon being the main source of life on this planet.
SEKHEM 'Absolute energy' commonly named prana or chi the active principle of life or vital life force.
SEKHEM is the name the ancient ones used for the universal principle which principle is the essence of all motion, force energy whether manifested in electricity, magnetism or the revolution of the planets from the highest to the lowest moving through out all of nature in all forms SEKHEM is the active universal principle also known as the soul of force. It is that form of activity that accompanies all life.
SEKHEM is in all forms of matter yet it is not matter it is in the air yet it is not one of the chemical ingredients of the air. It is in the food we eat and it is the true nourishing substance of the food and it is in the water we drink yet not a chemical component of water it is in the sunlight yet it is not the heat or the rays of the sun. It is the energy in all these things, the essence and the carrier. Animals and plant life extract Sekhem from the oxygen. Say if we were to breathe in pure oxygen it would poison us, Sekhem is what gives us life.
SEKHEM is in atmospheric air but it is also where air cannot reach. Oxygen and carbon play important roles to the building blocks of life. Sekhem role is the personification and maintenance of life on a spiritual level also known as the plane of force.

All physical manifestations have a spiritual counterpart for example; you. If you were to get sick and had to lie up in bed. Your sickness would have manifested in the plane of force/spiritual plane first then trickle down into your physical being. The plane of force is your 'Black Print' commonly called blue print this is the mapping of your being. That's is why our Afrikan healers would work holistic meaning mind body and soul derived from **Ka** spirit, **Ba** soul and **Khat** body from the principles laid down by the great Master Amun-Hotep student of Tehuti. All things have this black print so when eating an apple it is not just the nutrition of the apple you are extracting but the SEKHEM which feeds the spirit as well as the body. This is why organic is so important these days because you cannot create sekhem in a laboratory like GM food, which is a cloning process.

The air is charged with SEKHEM. The ancient ones knew this so would breathe slowly, deeply and rhythmically. They were able to extract this energy from the air more easily than any other source. The practitioner knows that through practise of the science of breath they are able to store this powerful absolute energy in their nerve centres and use when needed, The miraculous powers of occultist is due to the fact that they are aware of Sekhem and intelligently store this as a clay home would store the heat of the noon day sun or a battery would store electricity ready to switch on at will. The Smai Afrikan healers where able to generate psychic capabilities, using sekhem stored in the energy centres and develop their latent abilities. They exude energy of vitality and a healing personality that often radiated strength and would be received as healing when anyone would come in contact with them. They would convey this on anyone they wished and this is now known as magnetic healing, Reiki healing and Sekhem healing. There are many who as such a personality but is unaware of their source of power.

Sekhem is also a symbol of power, this was a staff of office the word Sekhem literally means power, Sekhem also symbolises the stars and his found in paintings with Asar.

Respiration
Is the cyclic process of inspiration and expiration. It denotes continuance to do and live again and again.

Inspiration
As described earlier taking a breath is known as inhalation or *inspiration*.
On an esoteric level inspiration is a divine inhalation of creativity which Tamareans Ancient Afrikans call outformation. Where you get a download from the outmost~ sphere, coming outside of this planet and at times outside of this solar system.

It is also the drawing in of life-force Sekhem and the initiating of a life process.

Expiration
Described as the out breath or exhalation which is the freedom of illnesses, getting rid in order to renew. It is the motion of completeness where the cyclic line has been completed to create another circle.

With expiration comes deep relaxation where one becomes Asar prepared and ready to resurrect in this world or the next it does not matter to the smai/yogi as they are fully aware the cycle continues.

$4+6=10$ $1+0 = 1$ which is the one~ss of being also add a 0 to 1 and you get 9.

NINE to The 9th Power

9 is a sacred number used by the ancient ones it is also the highest number in the numerical system. All numbers after 9 repeat themselves for example 0 zero after nine becomes 0ne and a zero 10. Number one 1 after nine becomes one and one 11 and two become one and two 12 so on and so on until you reach 9 and you go back to zero again. Starting now with a 2. Two and zero 20, two and one 21 this continues until you reach 9 and then another zero is added. This multiplying by tens 10 prior to the Afrikan/Nubian moors who brought the concept of zero which is a cipher would have left the whole of Europe in complete ignorance as they where counting with sticks and bones called 'Roman Numerals'. The shape of 9 in itself is a 0 and a 1 joined. This is also a computer system 1 and 0 called binary.

The binary number system or binary number code is a system of numbers to base 2 using combination of the digits 1 and 0. Codes based on binary numbers are used to represent instructions and data in all modern digital computers, the value of binary digits being represented as on/off states of switches and high/low voltage in circuits. The binary system is taken from the Ifa the divination system of the Yoruba peoples of Ancient Nigeria who migrated out of the land of Khemet alongside many other families named the Akans during the multiple invasions of the Phoenicians, Greeks, and Romans and in the last 1000 years pale skinned Arabs.

The IFA is an Afrikan spiritual ethic that lays down that ones destiny can only be reached through utilising three principles

1. The divinatory processes left to us by the ancestors

2. Prescriptions of ritual and sacrifice to the spiritual dimensional beings whose forces impacts upon human development and evolution

3. The moral ethics to which humans must adhere in order to be victorious over oppressive human and spiritual forces.

(Ref The Handbook of Yoruba Religious concepts/Baba Ifa Karade)

The binary system as been said to be linked to the Chinese I Ching which is also a divination tool, however, research as shown that the Ifa is at least a thousand years older than the I-Ching and actually birthed it.
(Ref to Ancient Future/Wayne Chandler)

74

Looking at these systems I can also propose that Ifa gave birth to western technological communication through Morse Code and Telegraphy.

Morse Code an international code for transmitting messages by wire or radio using signals of short and long dashes called duration. The name comes from Samuel Morse who invented the telegraph.

NINE

Composed of all-powerful 3x3 it is the Triple Triad; completion; fulfilment; attainment; beginning and end; the whole; a celestial and angelic number; The earthly paradise. It is an 'incorruptible' number. Nine is also the number of the circumference, hence its division into 90 degrees and into 360 for the entire circumference. It symbolises the two triangles which in turn is a symbol of the male and female, fire and water principles

This symbol is Pythagorean for Nine. However, the ancient ones symbol is the Egyptian star of creation shown below where Pythagorus derived his symbol from.

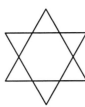
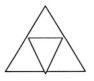

Egyptian star of creation became the 'Magen Dawid' Shield of David now known as the 'Star of David'.

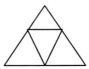

Pythagorus symbol for 9th to the 9th power

The average rate of respirations in human beings is 18 (=9) breaths per minute. In an hour, the average of course is 18 times 60 minutes, which equals 1,080 (=9) breaths.

In a period of twentyfour hours, one day, the average is 1,080 times 24, which equals 25,920 the time period of the Great Year. (The Great Year was known to all the ancient civilisations of the world and was first used in Tama-re KMT and in India. The ancient ones used this celestial clock to predict events way before they happened. The Tamareans Ancient Afrikans divided this great clock into 12 portions creating the zodiac)

As we breathe 18 breaths per minute the average pulse rate is 72 times a minute, seventy two is also the time it takes to transit one zodiacal degree in any of the twelve constellations. Seventy two pulses per minute equals 4,320 an hour. [The number of years in the Kali Yuga] our current epoch, is 4,320.

All the numbers equate to 9. (Ref Wayne B Chandler Ancient Future)

Dr Malachi Z York raised the awareness of the number 9 and taught extensively about its principles here is an example in 'The Holy Tablets'.

Holy Tablets Chapter 10
Disagreeableness, Tablet 11 'Nine Ether':
22-39

22. Universal knowledge, called Nuwaubu informs you, 'New Beings' that there were three creations:
23. Original or primary creation,
24. Evolutionary or secondary creation,
25. And Ghostational or tertiary creation.
26. Primary creation was performed by Nine ether whose science is Nuwaubu.
27. Nine ether is the combination of all existing gases of nature,
28. Thus, all is in The All.
29. Nothing anywhere can be as powerful as all existing gases.
30. Therefore nine ether is the most potent power in the universes, 9 –9th power of 9.
31. Nine is a very meaningful number, it is symbolic of heaven, hell and creation.
32. Nine is a number which is symbolic of the three dimensions.
34. Nasswut-abode of mortals
35. Malakuwt – abode of the Annunagi Aluhum
36. Laahuwt|- abode of The Most High; and
37. Nine is a number when multiplied reproduces the same figures from up to down and from down to up, and it equals itself.
38. Nine ether was placed in the follicle case of all original Nuwbuns, and it produces the 9 symbol.
39. When the number nine is inverted or perverted it becomes the number 6

9 creates 9 of itself no other number does this if you do your 9xtables you realise the power of nine. 9x1=9
9x2=18 1+8 =9
9x3=27 2+7=9

9x4=36 3+6=9
9x5=45 4+5=9
9x6=54 5+4=9
9x7=63 6+3=9
9x8=72 7+2=9
9x9=81 8+1=9
9x10=90 9+0=9

So it continues 9 is the infinite number of the universe and the sacred number of all Afrikans ("A free ka (ns") Tama-Reans ancient and modern. We are born from 9 Ether the originator of all existing gases, liquids and compounds.

Nine is the letter I [eye] in the English alphabet taken from the Greek alphabet also links into what is known as the A'IYN principle.

This is a sacred tone translated in Sanskrit as AUM

The 9 Enneads of Afrikan Yoga

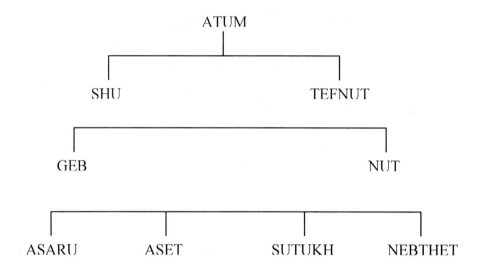

The nine eneads also know as the company of the deities of ANNU are the first beings created by Atum/RE.

The word Neteru has been translated as Gods and Godesses and deities this also equivalent to the Orisha of Yoruba, the Eloheem of Judaism, The Annunaqi of the Sumarians, the Allahum of Islam. These beings the Egyptians viewed as ones with great supernatural powers, yet where finite and mortal. These human deities were endowed with love, hatred and passions of every sort and many owned more than one title.

Shu
The Neter Shu "The Raise" according to cosmology of the people of Anu was created by a divine sneeze and was the Neter of the sky and the second member of the Ennead.

He was the first born of Ra/Re known also as the Neter of Air and Light also known as *'The Angel'*. He appears as a human with an Ostrich feather on top of his head and holds a sceptre in his hand. He is the twin brother and consort of Tefnut. There are times he appears in the form of man with his arms upraised.

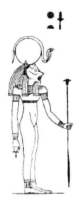

Tefnut
The Netert Tefnut is know as the the third member of the enneads she is the daughter of Re and the consort of Shu. Tefnut is symbolic of water in particular moisture not only all that is water but also the power of water. Tefnut is the form of a woman and a woman is symbolic of moistness and an internal creator due to her reproductive seat, her vaginal area as opposed to the male who is dry and a external creator. Water is the symbol of purification and personification as the first form of matter in all cosmologies. Tefnut is a lion Netert the symbol of courage and intuitive convictions and was worshipped as a lion, Tefnut and Shu in the form of Lions guarded the east and the west horizons Tefnut in another form personify as the power of sunlight.

Geb

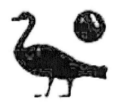

Or Seb is the Neter of the earth and as been known as the 'father of the deities'

Some times is depicted in human form with a goose on his head and because of the goose his symbol he is also known as 'The Great Cackler'. The sound the goose makes when giving birth and this is related to the story of baby being carried or brought to a family by a goose.

Nut
Nut is the female counterpart of Geb, and is the Netert of the sky and the the daughter of Shu and Tefnut. Nut has immersed the many attributes of Female Neters as they have close qualities and characteristics to her.

Set

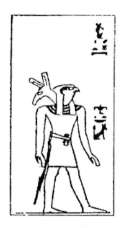

Or Sutukh was the Neter of Storm, night and drought. Sutukh is known as the promoter of illusions and his name gave birth to Set as in 'setting' sun which is an illusion as the sun neither rises nor sets. This leads into further misconceptions around darkness and light and good or bad which are flags waved fervently by religious doctrines.

This concept of darkness being bad is a very unhealthy ideology for Afrikans as they are the darkest people on the planet and this adds to our mental dis-ease.

Many of our scholars still refer to darkness as evil and this seems to be inbeded in our psyche by European education, religion and ideaology. This has to be unlodged as we can no longer afford to see ourselves as dichotomy but a harmonious whole. When you close your eyes are you in a state of darkness? Now in that state there is peace and true connection with your feelings, yourself and NETERU this means that the supreme beings and in deed The MOST HIGH reside in that state. So are you going to tell me that darkness is bad?

In the bible when God created light or said let there be light which means there was no light until it was said let there be light in what state was God in?

Yes in the state of Supreme Balance, darkness, triple Blackness (this is all light/true light not reflected light). Sutukh became Set the deity of night and darkness because of his rivalry with his brother this is the interpretation of the Greeks who stressed the rivalry story as they are well known for providing us with what is called The Greek Tragedy's which is your soap operas of today. We can see similarities in Enki & Enlil of The Gilgamesh Epics, Cain & Abel and Ishmael & Isaac, and Adonijah & Solomon of the bible and countless other brother to brother battles. This shows that most if not all ideas are based on Egyptian/Afrikan Mysteries. We all have this rivalry going on in our families so it is a very human story, however, Sutukh was exalted and chosen to ride on the bark of Ra as his defender against Apothis a serpent diety and promoter of ignorance, sleep, anxiety, fear and doubt. Sutukh who became Set and Seth in later times was synonymous with demons, evil, death and crime. Crime because it has been said that Set formed the first police state, during the absence of Ausir/Ausar/Osiris who ruled with benevolence, peace and justice.

Seth because this is associated with the language and names of the Hyskos 'Shepherd Kings' the invaders of Khemet who changed customs and rituals to suite their purpose and was viewed as malevolent. Sutukh according to the ancient ones is exonerated and a protecter Neter defender of Ra.

We neither see good or bad; we see what is.

Nephthys

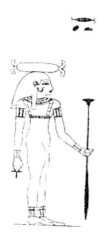

Known as Nebthet the consort of Set and the sister of Aset, her role as sister to Aset seem to place a greater value in the cosmology of KMT Ancient Afrika. Nephthys was very close to Asar and Aset. With Aset Nephthys was the protector of the dead and assisted Aset in finding the location of the 14 pieces of Asar. The goddess was also the mother of Anubis or Anpu fathered by Asar. A depiction of this story is that Nephthys in love and adoration of Asar went to his bed veiled and Asar thinking this was Aset slept with her and consummated Anubu. This is one of the reasons why Set filled with jealousy ('basically lost it') murdered is brother Asar. Nebthet is often shown as a woman with hieroglyph on her head that formed her name "Lady of the House".

Asar

Ausar/Asaru/Usir/Osiris, son of Geb and Nut.
The Neter of crops and vegetation and is often depicted as green. This is also due to his pure state as a cosmological being which contained less iron content in his body than most Nubians today. (Iron when in contact with oxygen and water turns to brown, rusts). Asar/Osiris is also known as *Lord of the Perfect Black*" this happens to be a title that Krishna of India carries. The Orion constellation is named after and associated with Ausar/Osiris.

Ausar is known as a solar deity and a pre-dynastic pharaoh of KMT who became the ruler of the dead and the underworld after his murder his body was re-membered by Aset/Auset which formed the first mummy. He is the equivalent to God the father and Jesus of the Christian faith, Isa of Islam and Tammuz of the Summerian doctrine (Ancient Babylon doctrine). He is often absorbed into attributes of other Neters and their attribute into his. He is the Neter of death, resurrection and fertility as this links into the decay, renewal and rebirth of crops. He taught his subjects how to grow barley and brew beer and ruled KMT with peace and justice; to that aim he travelled far and wide into other lands. He is mostly famed for the story of his death and members of his body being scattered throughout the land, gathered and placed together by his widow Aset. Who then aroused him sufficiently to be impregnated and conceive Heru/Horus who avenged his father and reclaimed rulership from Sutukh/Set.

Ausar has many forms and other 100 names too much to mention here, he is often seen has a green man in the form of a mummy wearing a crown and holding in his hand a crook and flail the emblems of sovereignty and power.

There are certain ceremonies today disguised as Easter which are ceremonies for Ausar. There is of course the opening of the mouth ceremony which is performed on the mummy of a pharaoh by the heir to legitimise the inheritance and this included purification, anointing and incantations in order to restore the right-mind.

Aset

Aset/Auset/Isis is the female consort to Asaru/Ausar the daughter of Geb and Nut and is known throughout Egypt and many cultures as a wise, nurturing lover and mother. The deity Aset is often referred to as 'The Divine Mother' or 'Mother of the Deities', 'The Living One' she usually takes on the form of a woman with a seat or throne on her head a hieroglyph of her name.

This Netert is known as Isis (wisdom) amongst the Greeks who also relate her to their deities Demeter, Selene and moon Goddess Astarte (star). In Sumeria she is known as Ishtar and Dina. Aset is Maya in Buddhism, Fatimah in Islam and Mary in Christianity. In the bible she is mentioned as Ashtoreth meaning star 1 kings 11:5 and 11:33. Aset or Auset or Eset iconography is often that of a mother suckling her child Heru/Horus. Who is the original image of the Madonna and child, Jesus and Mary image of Christianity. Asar, Aset and Heru are also The Holy Trinity. Aset is known as the deity with many names and is in all forms of female deities in particular Hathor whom she has borrowed the cow horns and indeed her sacred animal is also the cow and Maat where she is also depicted at times with wings and also the deity Nut. Aset fame is of her undying love for Ausar and her courage and protection of her son Heru that spread far and wide becoming a story of legend. Aset was worshiped and revered by the Romans and the Greeks and many temples were built in her name. She was highly skilled in the healing arts and known to pass on her knowledge to the people of the Nile. She ruled with wisdom and justice while Ausar travelled the world to spread peace. This made Set jealous has he thought himself a more fitting ruler than Aset.

When Set had cut the body of Asar/Osiris into 14 pieces and thrown them into the Nile. The dedicated Aset searched for each piece with the aid of Nephtys recovering all parts but the phallus that was swallowed by a fish.

This is all after Aset had travelled far and wide to find the body of Asar who was murdered and his body locked in a sarcophagus the trunk of a great tamarisk tree by Set. She eventually found the Tamarisk tree as a pillar in Lebanon, Byblos at the Palace of the king and Queen of that country, who had found the enchanting tree floating in the Mediterranean Sea. Auset brought Asar body back to Khemet were she used her magic to revive Asar so that she could be impregnated by him as he did not have an heir via their royal union and an avenger for his murder. This great ancestor Netert was also known as the Mistress of Charms and Enchantment and was able to obtain the secret name of Ra her Grandfather this increased her powerful magic. This was a true power move as Ra did not give the name away lightly even at the face of certain death. Aset was able to pass this secret name onto her son Heru, as Ra made her promise that he was the only one she could reveal his secret name to.

Heru

Heru/Hor/Haru/Horus is the famous falcon headed Neter who avenged is father Ausaru His depiction as a falcon or falcon headed man is linked to meanings around his names "on high", 'the distant one", and "far away" as well as being a solar deity who is the Jesus of Christianity, and Tammuz in ancient Babylon the holy son of God. Heru struggled and fought is uncle Set to avenge his father and to reinstate the rulership placing it back in to balance. The story of the wicked uncle or the avenging son is found in many cultures today even in cartoon movies like 'The Lion king' which is the Heru story. This battle was fought for many days and was a contest of strength, wit and nerve. In the battle Heru lost an eye that had to be restored by Tehuti and Het-Heru Hathor known as the Wedjat. However, this is the contest we undergo in our being as the Heru/ Hero.

Nine Principles of the Hueman Being

abdur kull tafulataat wa baazun amma faruⴰun shil el kuluwm

Abdur Kull Tafulataat Wa Baazun Amma Farugun Shil El Kuluwm
Begin All Prayers And Thinking As Apart Of The All.

ane baruf tased:
Ane baruf tased:
I know nine:

el tased kanruhaat:
El tased kanruhaat:
The nine principles:

ka, haza izu el nafuslal nee
Ka, haza izu el nafuslal nee.
   1. Ka, this is the spiritual me

khu, haza izu el aƋlu nee.
Khu, haza izu el a'glu nee.
   2. Khu, this is the mental me

khat, haza,izu el Ƌisum nee.
Khat, haza,izu el gisum nee.
   3. Khat, this is the body me.

ba, haza izu el rawuh nee.
Ba, haza izu el rawuh nee.
   4. Ba, this is the soul me.

khaybet, haza izu el khashuhik nee.
Khaybet, haza izu el Khashuhik nee.
   5. Khaybet, this is the plasmatic me.

84

```
akh, haza izu el atherik nee.
```
Akh, haza izu el atherik nee.
    6. Akh, this is the etheric me

```
hati, haza izu el maduy □alb shil lanee
```
Hati, haza izu el maduy galb shil lanee
    7. Hati, this is the physical heart of mine,

```
ab, haza izu el nafuslal □alb shil laka,
```
Ab, haza izu el nafuslal galb shil laka,
    8. Ab, this is the spiritual heart of yours,

```
sekem, haza izu el rame□ shil hayuh shil laka,
```
Sekem, haza izu el rameg shil hayuh shil laka,
    9. Sekhem, this is the spark of life of yours.
Taken in part from the Gold Book; The Sacred Tablet of Tama-re authored by
Ammonubi Ruakhptah.

The nine principles of the human being that corresponds to the supreme beings,
the Enneads, reside in us.

SEKHEM spark of life AMUN RE
AB spiritual heart of mine SHU
HATI physical heart of mine TEFNUT
AKH etheric me GEB
KHAYBET plasmatic me NUT
BA soul me ASARU
KHU mental me ASET
KHAT physical me SUTUKH
KA spirit me NEBTHET

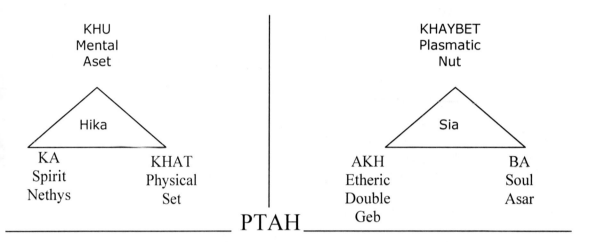

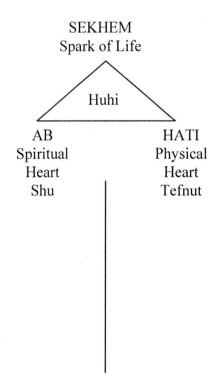

The diagram displays the 3 abodes of Huhi, Hika, physical realm Sia.

The 9 principles are interwoven through creation, which is why human beings unaware are interconnected with the principle deities through out time space and dimensions. They reside within us as us. Though there true power lays dormant within us a waiting for the spark through breath and tone to enliven us once again and bask in the rays of the (awareness) Sun

Ptah use the utterance of tone to create through HUHI this tone is known as AUM which became KUWN or KUN as in *kun faya Kun* spoken of in the Koran.

1. In order to create something the Neteru, who are also known as The Ancient Ones headed by, a group of RE called ATUM-RE, ATUN-RE AMUN- RE created a state of nothingness, in which to place 99 elements or attributes of this state by HU, Huhi, the eternal or things or things on this side of H₁.

"The Sacred Records Of Neter: Aaferti Atum-Re" (Amunnubi Ruakh Ptah) Chapter 1. 'The Coming': Scroll 3.

*296. In Egypt, **Huhi,** which is considered the personification of "utterance", with which the creator **Ptah "Ta",** who was regarded as the creator of the physical world and deity of technology done its work.*
*297. **Hu** was the utterance or tone, the vibration and pulsation of existence and that which comes to existence within the sacred breath.*
*298. Those things made, that manifest within creation, true growth, **Hu** is that tone from which the creator calls into being, with **Hika** and **Sia.***
*299. The original triad of **Ptah, Hika and Sia**. Huhi is one of the creative forces of will that constantly accompanies, **Re, "Ra",** the sun deity, the source of life, the provider of sustenance in this world, the eternal.*
*300. This highest triad is the triangle with the eye of **Re** in the centre, and the three points of the triangle represents **Atum** "the undifferentiated one", in the creation.*
*301. The full disc appearance of the sun in the morning **Atun** "the unique one" in life.*
302. The full sun disc at the highest point of the day.
*303. **Amun** "the hidden one", at death, sun at its last full disc before setting, and making it through the underworld or netherworld.*
*304. These are the sacred names of the three suns **Shamash, Afsu** and **Utu** of Sumeria, and **Hu. Huhi, Huwa**, is the etheric counterparts of the Nether world.*
305. These beings once dwelled in this realm and now they are guiding forces and controlling forces from beyond this world, working as the involuntary, to the voluntary in the human body.

"The Sacred Records Of Neter: Aaferti Atum-Re" (Amunnubi Ruakh Ptah) Chapter 1. The Coming': Scroll 1. 296-305.

Maulena Karenga who selected and retranslated the sacred wisdom of Ancient Egypt, coined the work THE HUSIA, which has the two principles HU and SIA placed together.

"The title of this text, The Husia is taken from two ancient Egyptian words which signify the two divine powers by which Ra [Ptah] created the world i.e, Hu, "authoritative utterance" and Sia, exceptional insight. Thus, I have put the two together to express the concept "authoritative utterance of exceptional insight". Given the importance of authoritative utterance of exceptional insight to the moral and spiritual realm of their divine character in ancient Egyptian theology, Husia appears as both compelling and proper as a title for a text of ancient Egyptian sacred writings".

From the introduction of THE HUSIA by Maulena Karenga

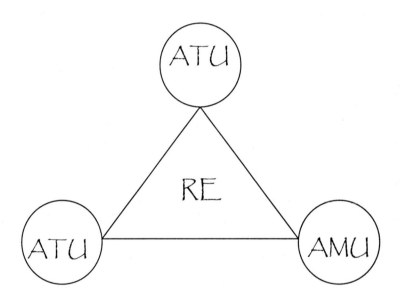

The Three States of Re, Atum "the undifferentiated one", Atun "the unique one" and Amun "the hidden one".

306. **Hika** is an anthropomorphic personification of miracles, magic, and the manipulation of elements, and chemicals of nature.
307. **Hika** is one of the two constant companions of **Re**. The other being **Sia**.

308. **Sia** is the personification of perception, shape form, pattern who work together in **Huhi** with **Hika** and makes the world of created things possible.

309. So, **Huhi**, **Hika** and **Sia** are a triad principle of godship, the Neteru responsible for the consistant and perpetual pattern of that which manifest, in that which is created, and made and that tone or utterance is Aum, which later was rendered as **Kun**, as in existence or **be**.

"The Sacred Records Of Neter: Aaferti Atum-Re" (Amunnubi Ruakh Ptah)

Chapter 1. 'The Coming': Scroll 1. 306-309.

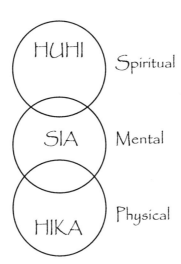

HUHI — Spiritual

SIA — Mental

HIKA — Physical

The 9 Purposes of Smai/Afrikan Yoga

1. Emancipation/Freedom

Freedom gives us the ability to really choose and not feel pressured into doing things that go against our spirit. You have freedom of expression and freedom of thought. Thinking for yourself, you are completely guided by your inner divine self and not manipulated by others. Some are bound by relationships some are bound by their guru or teacher. Freedom is when one merges into supreme consciousness and is "one with The All".

The practise of Afrikan Yoga is not only acknowledging freedom but to access freedom now in your life wherever you are in your life. It enables you to feel the wisdom of Maat flowing through your entire being be coming 'A Free Ka' (ka meaning spirit).

Many of us will now have to learn to be free, we may find it difficult, painful and unattainable. You can be free, by being true to yourself.

2. Action

"Do or Do Not, there is No Try" -Yoda, Star Wars.

Earlier I mentioned Maat and her divine principles. One of the key principles of Maat is that of action. Even though we may have gained intellectual knowledge and understand the maxims; repeat chapter and verse verbatim which in today society's may seem to be acceptable criteria for establishing a group or accepted by a clique.

Experience is the master teacher, which is one of the points of Nuwaupu the science of all nine ether solar beings (Tama-Reans /Afrikans).

It has to be understood that there is knowledge without thoughts and words; knowledge so abstract that it cannot be taught, only experienced, lived and breathed. The student and the teacher become one in the realisation of witnessing this knowledge that is much more than the intuitive self.

Within application, keen observation, perseverance, patience and compassion for oneself will this knowledge begin to reveal itself. The essence of this knowledge, is waiting for you, and constantly placing opportunities in our paths to grasp its spirit, to be it, to acknowledge and to express it and to know it. The opportunity arrives in the forms of near death experiences, trauma or witnessing trauma or even overwhelming joy.

The ari-action in Afrikan Yoga is fundamental it just goes without saying as I have been taught. *"Lift up the self by it self for the self is the self's only friend and the self is the self's only foe"*. Within this teaching you find yourself ultimately responsible for self and a recipe for self-mastery through action. Ari, the word for Action, is a principle of Maat in line with karma. In Afrikan Yoga, the principle of **Ari** is simply applied as a series of one or more exercises ragulaat (ragul) or postures *sayunaat* in combination with smai breath, gaanum (chanting), istanizaah (visualisation), and transformation, etc in specific sequence designed to produce specific effects. The ari-aat used in Afrikan Yoga (**Tamare Smai**) are thousand of years old. The effects of Ari are greater than the sum of its parts which is to say these sayunaat as simple as they look are not to be underestimated for their power to heal physically mentally and spiritually.

3. Knowledge

"If Knowledge is the key, then ignorance is the door" Khonsu Sekhem Ptah

"The purpose of acquiring knowledge is to nourish one's character. But one who merely pursues knowledge as an end in itself misses the point of education"
    Cai Gen Tan/The Vegetable Discourses by Hong Yingmin of the Ming Dynasty

"Know thy self" is the axiom of the ancient ones written on thy pylons of ancient Egypt this is an important part of Smai as knowing oneself is self-empowering.
    Many people have accepted "book learning" as the total sum of knowledge or method of knowing. This is unfortunate because knowing self is true knowledge because it is the means by which you perceive yourself as the microcosm of the boundless universe. Through meditation you learn this self-awareness this perception and you begin to project from within out. As apose to gathering of facts etc you develop insight. Through meditation you realise that you can turn yourself inside out creating your reality. The universe provides for you as you are the universe. Another axiom is *"As within so without"*.

4. Power

Those with true power have no need to flex their muscles as true power is a magnetic force that commands respect by its' sheer grace, serenity and influence. It is a manifestation of Sekhem that resonates in all aspects of your life. As I mentioned earlier many believe the idea of power as a big muscle bound male or acts of violence. Power exists in your self-image and therefore is a force of spirit. For the martial minded amongst you hear the words of Carlos

Castenada *"Warriors are in the world to train themselves to be unbiased witnesses, so as to understand the mysteries of ourselves and relish the exultation of finding what we really are".* What Carlos his actually speaking about is freedom and with freedom there is power as the two are synonymous. The suggestion is that a true warrior is liberated or free. It is this freedom that gives the warrior power. Warriors must purposely seek change.

The smai practitioner is a spiritual warrior and the ultimate realisation of the spiritual warrior is to flow into wholeness. This flow is with humility and transcendence that which is personal.

Personal power or acts of empowerment
Afrikan Yoga/Tamare smai assist the process of reclaiming your power by involving you in self-reliance through these steps.
1. Acceptance of self and who you really are and for you too overstand your issues and manipulations
2. Awareness and acceptance of your life and what you have created.
3. Acknowledge and appreciate your gifts, talents and abilities from the core and to separate this from the satellite superficiality that clogs your progress.
4. Be responsible for your life and no longer sit in a pain body being a victim and blaming others.
5. Pro-actively self-healing and seeking further changes in your life. The very reason that YOU do this, your life transfers into another level of personal power living free from, victim patterns and actualising your free will.

5. Love
Ashug/Love is represented by Hathor/Het Heru.
Ashug is a synergy, a glow that we feel; it's a light that reflects off of us. It's not something that we can use, its something that uses us. WE do not make love, create love, nor can we do these things, the best lovers are the vessels of love. The love that we feel is actually the connection to all things from all things. Ashug is the interwoven thread from the supreme conscious right down to the unconscious but when we are in a state of unconsciousness this love appears as something that we own, deserve and barter with and if things do not go our way this perception of love turns to hate. Actual ISHQ/ASHUG awakens you to your spiritual higher senses where one sees with an inner seeing, hear with an inner hearing and feel with the inner heart/spiritual heart. The lover accepts what is and with acceptance there is no resistance, no pain and no conditioning. "The All is I am" This is a person who carries light and rays of sunshine about their being they heal by just being present. Ashug is fundamental to the practitioner of smai without this purpose he/ she is an empty vessel. When we open ourselves up to

love we receive abundantly what the universe has to offer us. The universe is father/mother to us all. When we open up to the universe and universal love we begin to receive the guidance and assistance to pass through the "bottle necks" and "needles eyes" of life with ecstasy and ease.

6. Transcendence

"A person is said to be established in self-realization and is called a Yogi or mystic when he is fully satisfied by virtue of acquired knowledge and realization. Such a person is situated in transcendence[7] and is self-controlled. He sees everything-whether it be pebbles, stones or gold- as the same".

(Bhagavad-gita 6.8)

Afrikan Yoga/ Smai is a tool for developing transcendence moving from one state to the next mentally as spoken about in the HaKa the Hermetical laws of polarity, vibration etc. You gain transcendance through expression not repression.

That is to say the road to transcendance is not a self-rightous priesthood road where one pushes down their feelings, lusts, anger, jealousies etc, but by expressing these feelings and going into them deeply and purely. Once these feelings are experienced and explored they can be left behind, transcended. Transcendance is the complete awareness of illusion and not feeding into the illusion created by the ego. In a state of detached observation you rise above or move from so called problems, challenges and hurdles; reassigned to a state of higher consciousness, free from constraints and reactionary behaviour that often habituates your life moments and events. Transcendence is not being a person full of airs and graces with an attitude of 'I am' above you, or placing yourself as a judge of others, recognising the divine in all people. *"A person is said to be still further advanced when he regards all – the honest well wisher, friends and enemies, the envious, the pious, the sinner and those who are indifferent and impartial- with an equal mind".* (Bhagavad-gita 6.9). You see all as one and these labels cease to exist. Why because you know through your own experience. You are rooted and grounded in self-acceptance, self- love and your spirituality and therefore free to allow yourself to be. When truly accepting comes with allowing others to be also, no longer feeling the need to control their lives but allowing yourself and others to experience life as it unfolds. In the form of transcendence you become a Heru who is able to control his lower nature (ignorance, hate, jealousy etc,) and become one with his higher self 'Asar' one who is able to

---

[7] Transcendence is also the ability to see things as they really are.
Please refer to the 10 Virtues of Maat **'Learn to distinguish the real from the unreal'**

resurrect from a dead state of ignorance to a state of eternal life on the djed pillar of wisdom. This brings a state of hetep/peace.

7. Wisdom

"Wisdom is often found in the chambers of meditation". Khonsu Sekhem Ptah

The smai adherent looks to Tehuti (the male principle of wisdom) and Maat (the female principle of wisdom) in meditation and within their internal structure and within their bones and bone marrow where the DNA of our ancestors are kept.

This is the intuitive knowing when one says "I feel it in my bones". In combination with this knowing the 'Ari' action(s) of the aspirant is the personification of wisdom. Wisdom is not merely the manifestation of inspirational words and truth. It is also the divine, inspirational actions of truth that promotes harmony.

We are in a time of much devastation and ill will, however, the age of ignorance and destruction, the spell of sleep is lifting. The sleeping giant within us is awakening and the principles such as wisdom are now being activated to bring forth the supreme balance of Black Light that covers the full spectrum of waves, colours, moods, dimensions and realms. For all sit in Blackness even this planet is surrounded by Blackness. You know this once you venture out of this atmosphere, you know this once you close your eyes in meditation and feel the comforting nurturing womb of the universe expandng into nothingness into Pa Tempta The All. This is the realisation of the wise that *'nothing is all things'* a complete cipher to which you are apart, interconnected and one with ALL. Through meditation you may say I am not this body, I am not this thought or action. There is no identification with 'things' and this where you become nothing, interconnected to all things and vessel for the manifestation of the divine. It's a paradox. Have you ever asked someone what they are thinking after a break in conversation and they say 'nothing'. One or two things may be happening. One they have drifted in to subconsciousness. Two, they are unaware of the many thoughts that posses them. They are unable to slow down the process through feeling and then to communicate it clearly, conscisely and honestly devoid of judgement with love. The type of love we equate when a parent instructs a child. This wisdom is intricately linked to feminine values and once tapped used in all relationships. So when they express their thoughts it is authentic and self-aware.

8. Joy

Joy is a feeling of relief, of abundance, of achievement, of love, of heat that rises up your spine and fills the well of consciousness that expresses itself in a smile, in laughter, in tears and also in silence. Joy must be in all actions that you do, whether it is work, play or relaxation. When you do things joyfully you find that the task is effortless. Where there is no joy or enjoyment you will soon find a reason to stop. A person can perform a work or do their job joyfully with very little pay as long as they find joy in the tasks they will stick to it. A person can receive high amounts of pay for a job and not enjoy the job. They will soon give that job up or endure it painfully. Joy is a motivating force that will manifest abundance. Be joyful in all things.

9. Truth

"The Truth shall make you free" is a statement of: once you have dropped the dead weight of lies then you are able to soar to heights beyond your expectations. Truth does the miraculous work of laser cutting and healing. There is also recognising truth as a resonance of healing, why should one feel pain when they hear or see or feel truth, pain comes about through resistance of what is. In a Sanuy/posture your body does not lie it knows its limits in the now and it places you directly with now. (You may visualise yourself doing amazing things with your body; in your moment of now, the truth is the body will do a fraction of the things that you visualise, this is ok, keep visualising as your present truth will eventually change in due time). The Smai/Afrikan Yoga student learns to recognise truth through practical experience and not just as an intellectual experience of movement and form. This in turn applies to your recognition of truth in your daily life where you feel as well as observe and analyse. The continued practise then becomes more feeling and the fluidity of truth now begins to flood your being. There is now a synapses jump from the analytical I want, I need but I can't have. To spirit, feeling and I know, I have and I am abundant. With this awareness there is hope for future expansions on any dimension you wish. For truth in no way should way heavily on your heart. Truth sets you free.

Afrikan Seats of Light... The 9 Arushaats Cha ka ra(s)

The Arushaats (seats) in the body are focal points of exchange where the psychic, spiritual and physical planes of existence entwine to produce an exchange of energy. They work as transformers changing the subtle sekhem into physical energy that flow through the meridian lines in and out of these seat, connected to our personal atmosphere or energy field known as your Aura. Auras are called "Tepi Hesp" by the ancient Afrikans. The arushaats act as vortexes, whirlpools of great energy and they are 9 in total in the Afrikan and not 7 as which we are taught by the Indian Hindu yogis. The melanated Afrikan can perceive cosmic, gamma waves right down to radio, T.V. and electric waves in fact the whole light spectrum where Caucasians perceive the light spectrum of the rainbow which is 7 bands, also known as the visible light spectrum or standard photon band. Therefore the highest attainment of Caucasian body type is 7 chakras but really only attain 6. The reason is that the 7 bands or visible light spectrum placed in prism will breakdown into 6 colours. This is in line with the body type. The perception of the visible light spectrum and the electromagnetic spectrum is interlinked with the arushaats and melanin.

Arushaats Connection To Melanin
Melanin from mela means black. Afrikans are not taught about melanin in school. This would empower them to think for themselves and indeed to perceive their dark skins as an asset rather than a liability. Therefore opening their minds to their own divinity and seeing themselves as living sun entities very aware of life, and their connection to the universe. The subject of Melanin is key to the understanding of Afrikan spirituality, chakra activitiy and capabilities that appear to be superhuman and even supernatural. Dr Carol Barnes, Dr Llaila o Afrika, Jewel Pookrum and Richard King speak intensively on Melanin and their works studied with fervour will serve you well in the understanding of Melanin and indeed the understanding of the A Free Ka (n) people.

Carol Barnes tells us in his introduction to the book **Melanin: The Chemical Key to Greatness…**

"The Black Human is blessed by nature in that he or she is endowed with a highly functional chemical that regulates essentially all bodily functions and activities. The Black Human is distinguished from other human species in that he or she tends to have higher number of organs and body systems that contain high concentrations of a chemical that is BLACK in colour. This Chemical is called MELANIN and is responsible for manufacturing and sustaining life.

MELANIN is located in important areas of the BLACK HUMAN such as:

> *Central Nervous System*
> *Autonomic (Automatic) Nervous System*
> *Peripheral (outlying, surface) Nervous System*
> *Diffuse Neuroendocrine (Glands) System*
> *Visceras (Major Internal Organs)*

Because of it's pervasive presence in the organs, nervous systems and glands cited above, you would expect MELANIN to serve some vital function, or nature would not have incorporated it into these systems!

What Carol Barnes is saying in this last statement is MELANIN is key to the bodily system of all people on the planet as it is more prominent in Afrikans; western scientist are not raving about it and have suppressed it's information as a vital function and this is hideously amazing hence the exclamation marks.

There is much more to be said about melanin however, I want to direct you to the Arushaat/ (C)ha-ka ra (s), the connection to melanin. Why Afrikans have nine and why I have mentioned that Afrikans perceive higher states of consciousness naturally. Melanin is a key component in the ability to do and actualise this.

Blackness is all light and all energy and indeed absorbs all light. You only have to read and listen to scientist has they explain Black Holes. The study of photography and chromatics can also explain this, as the subject of photography teaches you about light spectrum and colours, which are forms of energy that are percieved.

Carol Barnes explains this *eloquently: "MELANIN is BLACK simply because its chemical structure will not allow any type of energy to escape once that energy has come into contact with its structure". Carol Barnes goes on to say The Human eye sees the colour of an object as light reflects from the surface of that object. If no light or energy is reflected, then that object will appear to the eyes to be BLACK in colour. If all of the energy is reflected from the surface of an object, that object will appear white in colour.*

If an object appears red in colour then that object is absorbing all energy around it except the red energy which is reflected away from the object.

Light energy from the sun or artificial sources like your indoor light bulb or vibrational sounds from your stereo, all causes melanin to be black in colour, for instance a light wave leaves the sun or your stereo in the form of enegy particles and/or vibrational sounds and travels in space until it contacts the melanin structure in your skin, and other areas of the body where it is absorbed by MELANIN".

Melanin: The Chemical Key to Greatness

This is to say that we not only perceive energy through the human eyes. According to scientists who now attest to what the ancients have taught that we are made up of fine particles of energy that are constantly vibrating and this is the make up our bodies, our skin, (skin colour and tone) limbs, organs and glands.

Corroborating this with Carol Barnes research it is suffice to say Afrikans are absorbing and perceiving (not reflecting) high amounts of light, colours, sound and wave lengths of energy. Making them darker in pigmentation but also giving them access to higher states of energy through the photon or visible light spectrum. The visible light spectrum perceived by Afrikans covers electric power, radio, T.V, micro-waves, infra red. Other frequencies of light perceived by Afrikans are ultra-violet, x-rays, gamma rays and cosmic rays. This is interlinked with glandular activity alongside the Arushaats. (Seats of light within the body). Note Afrikans of dark pigmentation must beware that this is a manifestation of outer melanin that makes up colour and there are thousand other forms of melanin within the body, with chemical, physical and personality properties. This is not an opportunity to tell yourself that you are superior to anyone else. Lighter skin Afrikans also posses the uniquness melanin gives. Europeans may be deficient in melanin yet some use the little they have to greater effect than Afrikans. There is also the problem of Afrikans becoming sick because of the melanin becoming toxic due to inadequate diet, lack of exposure to sunlight, detrimental music and thoughts. The quality of melanin is related to lifestyle and spiritual practise.

"The black dot is an ancient symbol for blackness, it is the black seed of humanity, archetype of humanity, the hidden doorway to the collective, unconsciousness-darkness, the shadow, primeval ocean, chaos, the womb, doorway of life".

Dr Richard King, African Origin of Biological Psychiatry

"The circle is the symbol of the crown Chakra. The circle sometimes contains a single black dot to indicate the first principle, the source of existence. The circle represents spirit and the whole cosmos, everything that is. The dot is the seed of a new life, the limitless given form".

Cassandra Eason, Chakra Power for Healing and Harmony

The sekhem the ancient name for energy that flows through the meridian channels is assisted by melanin that allows the energy to flow fluidly easily absorbing and conducting energy. The Afrikan smai practitioner uses this knowledge to fully engage in what is happening. Utilising this in their psycho-physical states the Afrikan yogi transforms themselves at will and converse with the ancient Afrikan scientists the Neteru who emerged out of Blackness and were the first to study and clearly understand the principles of the universe. They did this by studying their own Blackened state a methodology they leave with us today for we are told to "Know thyself". We can do this by studying the outer and inner blackened state, inner state through meditation.

The 9 arushaats overlap and feed into each other. They also represent the various dimensions of existence. Within the chart are placed glands of the endocrine system which effect growth, nerve action.

The 9 Arushaats (c)ha ka ra(s)
Table:

Arush	Location	Organs/glands	Symbolism, dimensions, existence	Colours
9.Ikh Ether	Head	Pineal	Mental/Meditating	White/Black
8. Mer Spirit	Brow	Hypothalamus	Intellect/Thinking	Violet
7. Shiru Breath	Nasal	Pituitary	Air Life Breathing	Indigo
6. Sehem Mucous	Throat	Thyroid/Parathyroid	Protecting/Verbal Communication	Turqoise
5.Heper Blood	Heart	Thymus	Healing/Curing	Green
4. A'b Solar Plexus	Diaphragm	Adrenals	Heating Circulation	Yellow
3. Tekhet Liquids	Navel	Islets of langerhans/Pancreas	Life Nourishing	Blue
2.Tchet Sacral Semen, Ovum	Groin	Ovaries/Testes	Carnal/Reproducing	Orange
1.Setekht Base Soul –E-motion	In between Perenium & base of spine	Prostrate/uterus	Lusting	Red

Personalities of Unbalanced and Balanced Arushaats/Energy Centres

SETEKHT Prostrate/Uterus

UNBALANCED
Insecure
Fearful
Feel unstable
Feelings of lack/Poverty conscious
Financial issues
Inability to let go and trust
Possessive
Disconnected from the environment
Feeling of isolation
Feeling drained
Ungrounded
Want to leave the body
Escapism

BALANCED
Secure
Feelings of abundance
Prosperous state of mind
Feeling safe
Ability to trust
Connected to the earth

At one with your body
Grounded

TCHET Semen/Ovum
UNBALANCED
Obsessive behaviour/including sexually
Inclined to jealousy and revenge
Dissected/separateness
Unable to satisfy creative expression
Unable to accept self
Crave what you feel you cannot have.
Inner child is in pain

BALANCED
Sexuality is integrated into your life.
Opportunities of creative expression are in every part of your life.
Connection with others
Love self
Secure in self
Spontaneous/flow with life
Healed inner child

TEKHET Naval
UNBALANCED
Anger
False pride
The need for recognition
Selfish motivation

BALANCED
Dissolved anger
Feeling of connection
No longer need to manipulate others
Self- importance fade
Positive ego identity
Selfless service develops

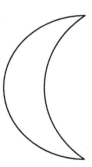

AB Solar Plexus

UNBALANCED

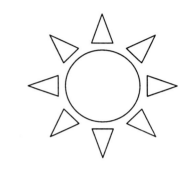

Not centered
Open to disease
Lack vitality
Inability to commit and maintain actions and intentions
Unable to break habits
Addictive
Possessive
Seek personal power
No consideration for the common good
Lack integrity and honesty
Revengeful and angry
Me first
Feeling of being a victim
A blamer

BALANCED

Centred
Vitality and health
Personal power
Wisdom and strength
Ability to commit, persevere and maintain
Flexibility/Ability to change
Reflect on inner sounds
Unattached
Ability to consider the common good
Integrity
Love and compassion radiate from within

HEPER Heart

UNBALANCED

Emotionally attached
Dependent relationships
Neediness
Selfish
Self-hate
Jealousy and envy
Weak immune system
Feel alienated from life

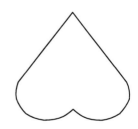

Sacred Spiritual Heart that points to
the divine

Lack of purpose
Depressed
Inner conflict

BALANCED
Male and female energies synchronised
Balanced relationships
Compassionate detachment
Self-love
Strong immune system
Ability to heal oneself and others
Committed to the universal plan
Contented
At peace

SEHEM Throat/Thyroid
UNBALANCED
Fear of communicating
Inability to express self
Delayed reactions
Hesitant in interactions

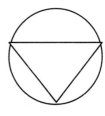

BALANCED
Ability to fearlessly communicate and speak one's own truth
Quick intelligent response
Self confident in interactions

SHIRU Nasal pituitary
UNBALANCED
Blocked creativity
Inability to sense danger
See no way out
Struggling with thoughts
Disorientated
Memory impaired

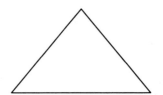

BALANCED
Clear thinking
Even clarity
Control of breathing and heart rate

Sensing energies
Open, alert and intuitive
Access memory and all dimensions of time

MER Brow/Hypothalamus
UNBALANCED
Have to analyse everything
Need physical proof
I believe it when I see it/ overly cynical
Fixed in mind and intellect
Non-accepting
Caught in emotional pain

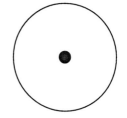

BALANCED
Intuitive knowing
Sensing abilities
Mind serves higher self
Inner hearing, inner seeing and inner feeling
Can listen inside and get an answer

IKH Crown/Pineal
UNBALANCED
Only aware of physical reality
Unable to move beyond the five senses
Distrust and negate (ancestral) higher forces
Have to take control
Do it alone mentality
Alienated from soul
Negate inner being

BALANCED
Experience realities beyond the physical preceptors of the five senses
Open to all realities of existence
Ability to perceive feel and experience soul
Ability connect to inner being
Trust higher powers

- *Only the well centred, well grounded and well balanced can dance, revolve and spin along and beautifully*
- *Real understanding lightens the heart*
- *Calm unshackles frenzy's grip*
- *Throughout the unfolding of each day, enlightened ones never lose touch with their inner-centre and transcendence*
- *Only when well rooted in the certainty of spiritual intuition can one realise freedom and transcendence*
- *You might well ask how anyone with responsibility can act without a sense of calm and understanding*
- *Inattention indicates instability*
- *Agitation indicates a loss of centre*

26 Tao Te Ching by Lao Tzu

Hekau

Word-Sound and Power

The Science of Sound

Healing

Holy Tablets Chapter 1: Tablet 7: 72-73

72. After a universe collapses in its centre or contracts, it expands, which is an explosion called: a "Big Bang", producing the sound KHA from which the word KHALUG 'create' comes.

73. It is the same sound that each being comes into this world, as the womb contracts to yield for birth, and the baby girgles GHA, and KHA, remembering the sounds of chaos in creation, as one thing comes into existence, it fractures other things to form itself.

TONES

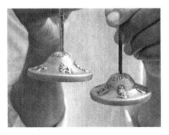

When you make a tone you summon forth light from the spinning wheels/Arushaats that are set in motions due to resonating sound to come and fill the corresponding organs with life, movement and revitalisation.

Afrikan Yoga movement and forms what we call **Hanu** and **Sanuyaat** are enhanced with the use of tones. The tones are used with the breath coming from the diaphragm up into the back of the throat and exhaled or expelled out to create the sound. In the Om or Ankh the sound comes from the diaphragm up in to the back of the throat exhaled out with the mouth slowly closing. Now the tongue is touching the roof of the mouth allowing the sound to vibrate into the nasal area. This links into Shiru arush opening the Mir Arush (third eye).

The 9 tones that corresponds to the 9 parts of the hueman.

A (pro nounced AAAAAH) a Healing and stimulating tone for the lymphatic system and digestion

AH (pro nounced AAAAAAUUUUUHHH) Healing and stimulating tone for the respiratory system

HAH (pro nounced HAAAAAAAAAHH) Healing and stimulating tone for the heart, gall bladder and liver.

KAH (pro nounced KAAAAAAAAAHHH) Healing and stimulating tone for the pineal, kidney and bladder.

E (pro nounced EEEEEEEEEEEHHHHH) Healing and stimulating tone for the pineal, the pituitary and nasal (*arushaat)*

O (pro nounced OOOOOOOOOHHHHH) Healing and stimulating tone for the pancreas and spleen.

U (pro nounced UUUUUHHH) U is a healing, stimulating tone for the stomach and large intestine.

OM/Aum (pro nounced AAAAAAUUUMMMMM)[8] Allow this tone to vibrate into the nasal cavities. OM is a healing and stimulating tone for the entire nervous system and all (*arushaat*) energy centres. Resonating from the solar plexus through to the nasal seat.

Ankh (pro nounced AAAAAAUUUUUNNNNNNNKHH) Allow this tone to vibrate into the nasal cavities. Ankh is a *healing, stimulating tone for the heart and life resonance on all planes.*

---

[8] Om/ Aum is also short for Amun this tone is used
(pro nounced AAAAAAAUUUUMMMMMUUUUNNNNNNN)

Hikau (Mantra) for Psychic Self-Defence and Transformation

Psychic Self-Defence.
Heru Wadjet Udjat heru wadjet udjat
"Calling on the all seeing eye of Horus".
Psychic attack of any kind; also for the promotion of strength and vigor.

Uplifting the consciousness.
Sa-Su-Temu – Heru-Hakenu sa-su-temu heru-hakenu
"Making an offering to the son, to Temu-Horus, the praised one"
To lift the consciousness into realms of mental and super mental activity that ranges far beyond the physical.

Immediate protection
Erta Na Hekau apen Aset erta na hekau apen aset
"May I be given the words of power of Isis"
Can be used to initiate immediate aid and protection it can also be used to provoke intuitive hints for action for anyone facing any form of threat, be it from physical danger or disease or of a psychic or spiritual nature.

Strength of Will and Purpose
Asaru –Djedu asaru – djedu
Incorporating the Djed principle. Used to promote strength of will, wisdom and overstanding also to nurture spiritual transformation and growth.

Happiness and Good fortune
Nefer Neter Wedineh nefer neter wedineh
"The perfect God grants life"
Repeating this attracts protection, inspiration, happiness, good fortune and a bonding with higher forces. It can also be used with a Neter's name drawing on the attributes of the chosen Neter.

Transformation from Human to Super Human Mantra
Ankh. ankh.
Tone: **AH UN KH A** (pro nounced AAAAAAAUUUUUUUNNNNKHHAAAA)

3 Names of Ptah.
Ankh Ptah Sekhet ankh ptah sekhet

Asaru asaru
For a protective force on all levels of human activity and a process of transformation from human to superhuman.
Tone: **A SAH RU (U)** (pro nounced AAAASAAAAAAHHRUUUUUU)

Pa Faatuh/The Opening
Hikau used to open the spiritual channels and raise the spirit in the abodes of the 3 suns ATUM, ATUN and AMUN. This hikau can be useful prior to, during and after meditation. This hikau can also be used before your practise.

Aum Atum Aum Atun Aum Amun Aum Kuluwm Aum

Amun
To Awaken the KA/spirit
Tone **AUM MUN** (pro nounced AAAAAAAUUUUMMMMUUUUNNNNNNN)

DIVINATION OF THE BODY MEMBERS

PRT EM HRU
PLATE XXXII

My Hair is of NU
My Face of RA
My eyes of HTHRU
My two ears of APUAT
My nose of KHENT-SHEPS
My two lips of ANPU
My teeth of KHEPERA
My neck of AST
My two hands of KHENEMU
My forearms of NEITH
My Backbone of SUT
My vagina of MUT (females)/My phallus of ASAR (males)

My thighs of KHERABA
My chest of SESEF-T-U
My belly and back of SERKET
My buttocks of the EYE of HRU
My hips and legs of NUT
My feet of PTAH
My fingers and toes of the LIVING ARAT-U [Urei]
Not a member of mine is without Divinity
TEHUTI is protecting my flesh entirely
I AM RA everyday... I come forth advancing
Seer of Millions of years is my name traveling along the path of HRU.
I feel... I perceive... I am in the UACHAT... I exist by its Strength
I come forth and I shine... I go in and I come to life... My seat is on my throne
I sit in the pupil of my eye by it... I have commanded my seat

I rule it by my mouth speaking and in silence
I maintain an exact balance season from season.
I Am, That I Am A Shining Being
Dwelling in (Black) Light, Dwelling in (Black) Light, Dwelling in (Black) Light
Dwelling in (Black) Light I Am.

Note: The words of a solar being

Afrikan Yoga and its Benefits

A prayer before a session
The Prayer of Asar (Osiris)

I fly up from you oh mortals
I am not for the earth
I am for the sky
I have soared to the skies,
I have kissed the skies as a falcon
I am the essence of deities,
The sun of deities,
The messenger of deities
I am in the light of Re
The light of Re is entering me
I am life itself

Warm ups/ Pa Raagus the dance and Hudu (Afrikan Tai-chi)

This is the symbol for Aker. The combination of Tefnut and Shu that signifies the horizon, the point where night turns to day, where day turns to night. This is depicted as two lions seated back to back, facing away from each other. They are also called Yesterday and Tomorrow, as one lion faces towards the east where the sun rises and begins the new day, the other lion faces west where the sun sets and descends into the Underworld. They protect the western and eastern horizons. Aker/Akiru also guards the gate to the Underworld and opens it for the King to pass through. According to a prominent Ancient Egyptian myth, the legendary 'gates of the afterworld', were guarded by two gigantic lions or sphinxes, called Aker/Akiru. In New Kingdom tomb drawings the aker-sphinx of the eastern gate sits proud with its hind parts in a hollow. Underneath it can be seen a curious underground stream or duct. Behind the lion towers a huge mound or pyramid and under it is found a large, oval chamber which appears to be hermetically sealed.

Most of the warm ups utilise Ka~Akiru' 'the spirit of the lion' ancient stretching techniques. Which has been formed from Netert Tefnut 'moisture' and Shu 'air' the two combined is known as HUDU (Afrikan Tai-Chi)

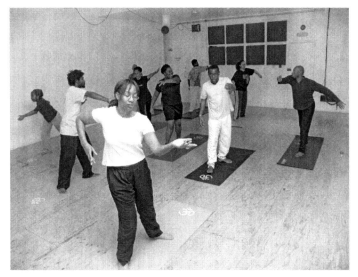

AIR & WATER
Holding the plates
Holding the plates is a fun way of stretching, utilising breath, imagination and dance. Stand upright with legs shoulder width apart. Turn your palms upwards keeping the fingers together and imagine that you are holding a plate on each hand with your dinner on it. Begin to reach forward and outward slowly at first guiding the plates around your body in sweeping movements twisting your torso inhale and exhaling deeply. Keep your palms facing upwards as the object is not to drop your plate.

You twist and turn your wrist in and out according to your movements avoid turning your palms down or sideways so not to drop your dinner.

Each stretch is precise and deliberate yet you flow like a summer breeze. Use your imagination, the more experience the more you become, the more you can stretch the legs and use balancing techniques etc, speeding up as your confidence grows.

Plant and Harvest
This movement or hudu looks like the jinga in capoirera and ngoma in kazimba. The first phase of this hudu is to stand upright with the legs wide apart and outstretch one arm further than the other. Twist the body side to side throwing one arm behind you and as you twist around lean back.

Once you have done this a few times using deep breathing, begin to sweep the floor lightly with both hands still twisting the torso in rhythmic movement building momentum.

The second phase is to continue sweeping the floor and now to rise up after each sweep twisting the torso, leaning back and throwing your arms back over your shoulder. This is an enactment of an Afrikan story of planting and harvesting where as you sweep you are picking vegetation and placing it in the basket on your back.

This warms up the spine, increasing the flexibility of the spine torso and works the legs, ankles and knees; develops concentration and rhythm.

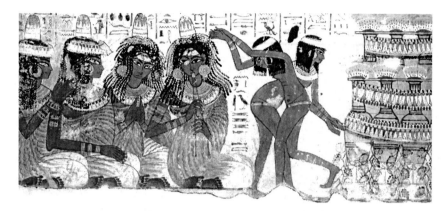

Pulling the boat of Re
Stand with feet wide apart and imagine you are taking hold of a rope by turning to the side and stretching out an arm, pull and exhale. Inhale, and then stretch out the other arm to continue pulling the rope. Begin to do this with a continuous stream of rhythmic movement, keeping the legs wide as you lean to grab, bend the knee facing the imaginary rope stretching the back leg. Change sides and pull there for a while, without stopping the flow of movement begin pulling from other directions above and below and from behind.

Swinging tree
The swinging tree utilizes side bends that stretch the torso, arms and hips creating greater flexibility in those areas and releasing anxiety.

Stand upright with feet together. Place one hand behind your back and the other arm and hand pushed straight up, let this arm rest alongside your ear. Inhale and lean towards the opposing side of the arm pushed straight up as far as you can and exhale and return to the position. Change arms and repeat the process.

The Practice
Guidance Notes:
1. Always warm up.
2. Never push yourself to the point of pain.
3. Always relax in between Sanuyaat/posture.
4. When in Sanuyaat use the breath.
5. When in Sanuyaat bear in mind the deity of the posture.

Yoga movements in particularly movements into extreme positions should be performed slowly. This is to ensure there is conscious control of the muscles; as in that jerky or rapid movements are not controlled and can result in an injury.

All yoga movements start with a ready position. This ready position preparatory breathing is carried out which is an inhalation and exhalation which is an initiation process for the movement.

Injuries in the joints or muscles are most likely to occur when the muscles are out of control either through jerky movements, speed, lack of breath or the incorrect approach to the movement

Pa Baagum Istamzaab "The Standing Position"
The standing position lengthens the whole body and re-establishes the balance of the body. In the standing position stand tall, keep the head erect, look straight ahead, the back is kept straight, the feet is slightly apart and the arms are hanged loosely by the sides that is considered to be the ideal position for a number of breathing techniques due to the fact that the distribution of muscular stress is fairly even throughout the entire body.

Breathe deeply into the abdomen and on the inhale push the stomach out. Exhale and draw the entire abdomen towards your spine.

Neck rolls
Unaat Humans carry a lot of tension in their necks, shoulders and upper back. Applying neck rolls before beginning Sayunaats/postures will help release the tension and blocked energy trapped in the neck, shoulders and upper back. You may do this either sitting in easy pose or standing erect where the body's weight is evenly distributed.

Eye of Re
ayun shil usa

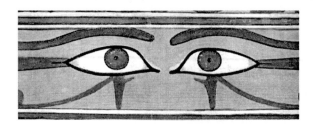

The Usa eye of Re is known as the all seeing eye. However, this eye is commonly referred to as the third eye the spiritual eye that perceives; views things, events and happenings in different dimensions and time. It is in reality the first eye. All seeing and all knowing this eye is the eye we possess linked to our divinity, especially at birth. When a new born arrives his or her third eye is open. If born in a hospital the doctors and nurses shine bright artificial light on the mother and child. These bright lights are a shock to a new born who has grown in a darkened womb and accustomed to seeing in the dark and perceiving things through touch, vibration and their third eye. The artificial light immediately causes an adverse effect on the child and the third eye begins to shut down and has to be reactivated through a DNA explosion. That is why in Ancient Afrikan culture we keep the child in a darkened room for days some times 10 days until the child grows more accustomed to its new environment where there is night and day and the third eye more or less remains intact.

In KMT the eyes are important symbols of Re, Asar and Heru in combination there power to see all is unlimited. The eye of Asaru is known as the **Utchat** this represents the sun and the eye of Heru is the **Udjat** which is a night eye/shadow or moon. Many confuse these eyes and are unaware that they're 3 with interchangeable attributes and many often refer to this eye as the 'evil eye' ignorant to the fact that the eye itself is not evil but the eye witnesses evil.

There are those who fear these eyes and teach the fear of them because they feel they are unable to do wickedness in the presence of the eye of Re as they will be seen and revealed. These eyes are superimposed on the brow arush and pineal gland. Heru was gifted the eye of Re when he lost one of his eyes in the battle with Set and this is why the eye of Heru is often refered to as the eye of Ra/Re.

"The pupil is the black dot. The portal through which light passes through the black doorway of the collective conscious. Blackness appears to be darkness (ignorance) to a Sethian lower mind consciousness. It evokes fear of the dense

material matter that cannot be penetrated by strictly logical mind. BLACKNESS or the VEIL OF ISIS (consciousness) does invite communication by the way of the heart, highly evolved feeling tone and intuition. It is this faculty of feeling tone, intuitive mind that is the hallmark of the Afrikan mind, immersed in symbolism and fluent in the language of time and space".

Dr. Richard King MD, African Origin of Biological Psychiatry

Eye exercises

The eye is brain tissue and links in with cognitive workings of the brain through the various nerve cells known as reticular formation. The exercise of the eyes assists the brain to be alert and balanced in the left and right hemispheres.

"Do not despise the body for it is the temple of the living spirit"

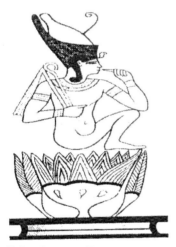

Sitting Sanuyaats for meditation

All of the various sitting positions for meditation are calming and nurturing; some promote the opening of the hips and require more effort. In general when practised properly with the spine and pelvis aligned they endorse a great deal of vitality, improving the circulation, reducing fatigue, soothing the nervous system and centring the mind.

These positions of meditation can be done at any time; however, the best times are in the morning after yoga practise when the body is warm and the limbs loose. Sitting will be easier and more welcoming as the mind will be focused and less cluttered with the days work. The positions are a recommended daily practise alongside your Afrikan Yoga/ Smai sanuyaat practise.

While in these positions you can also choose any "Taruh" hand position you wish or naturally require. (Please refer to Taruh Hand positions). You can use a pillow, cushion or folded blanket to sit on for comfort.

Pa Jaalus Istamzaab or The sitting Heru/Hero

The Sitting Heru sanuy or position is one form that most of us will be familiar with especially if you have been taught to pray or prostrate as a child as it involves kneeling and being still. This is also part of the final sequence of the *Ashutat* prayer positions and movements of the Egyptians. This position is known to Indian Yogis as 'The Rock'. The advance version of 'The Rock' in Indian yoga is still for Afrikan Yoga 'Sitting Heru' called the Hero.

The word hero comes from Heru or which the Greeks named Horus the falcon deity and the legendary hero of ancient Egypt.

From Horus we also derived the words, horizon, horizontal, hours and horoscope. Before attempting this make sure you can sit comfortably in this position for more than a minute. Make sure the heels are pointed straight up for correct alignment and knee protection.

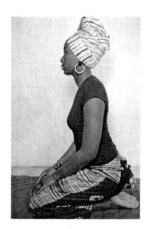

Start by kneeling on the floor with you buttocks comfortably on the back of your legs, feel your feet open to support your buttocks and slightly lift the knee to release tension from the knee caps, make the spine tall and place the hands on top of the thighs bring them slightly apart. Move the pelvis forward; sit for nine deep breaths.

For advance Heru your buttocks touch the floor with your feet folded straight back along your thighs. Breathe deeply into your abdomen for nine breaths.

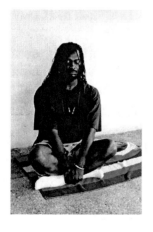

Easy Pose

This is for developing a positive and steady base for the body keeping the energy centred. When sitting in this pose you can use a hand taruh. The ancient positions of thumb and index or any other fingers or clasping the hands together in a interlocking position (Aset) or another alternative is place the hands in your lap one hand in the other. Easy pose calms the mind and relaxes the body in preparation for meditation. The position assists the opening of the hips and is a comfortable sitting position for meditation and breathing exercises.

Begin by sitting on the mat crossed allow your feet to rest below the knees

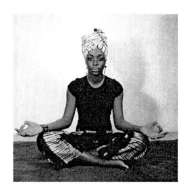

Nefertem "Beautiful Completion" (full Lotus)

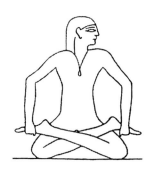

Kemetic Lotus

The lotus position is probably the most recognisable posture of yoga. From Buddha and Buddhism to Mystics and Sufism to Bruce Lee in the movie "Enter the Dragon" this posture is renouned the world over for centering and focusing the mind.

There is a prayer or request you can use in Nefertem for being transformed into the lotus taken from "Coming Forth by Day" Translated by AmunNubiRoakhPtah

1. O Lotus
2. Belonging to the semblance of Nefertum, *"The perfectly Beautiful",*
3. I am the Man
4. I know your names, you Neteru
5. You the Masters of the Neter's Domain,
6. For I am one of you.
7. May you grant that I see the Neteru's Domain, in the presence of the Masters of the West,
8. May I take my place that it desires,
9. Without being held back from the presence of the great Ennead (Nine Neteru)

ps. Inhale deeply and lengthen your spine drawing your shoulders back allowing the shoulder blades to gently slide closer, relaxing the shoulders.

Exhale and allow yourself to be rooted from your pelvic floor gently softening in to the pose. Relax breathing steady and rhythmically. Sit as long as you wish.

You may also use a hikau of Yaa Nefertem 24 times in the morning to develop youthfulness, enthusiasm and vigour.

Nefertem rising (Half Lotus or Adept posture)

This Sanuy is close to Nefertum (full Lotus) and is often called easy pose as it does not require both feet to be high on the thigh.

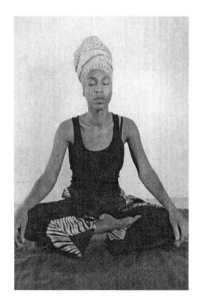

Sit with your legs extended in front of you make your The benefits are:

Physically

1. It opens the hips,
2. Increases knee flexibility and lubricates the knee joints
3. Prevent arthritis and osteoporosis
4. Tone the abdominal and encourages digestive functions

Mentally

1. Nefertem focuses the mind
2. Reduces stress and bring mental clarity

Do not use this pose if you have low back, knee or hip injuries. Sit with your legs extended in front of you make your spine tall by sitting up.

Draw one heel towards your navel and turn your foot and leg outward and place it on your lap at the top of your thigh. Draw your other heel towards your navel and turn the foot and leg outward placing them on the top of your opposite thigh.

Wrap your toes over your thighs flexing and pressing them down into your thighs.

Widen your thighs and hi spine tall by sitting up.

Draw one heel towards your navel and turn your foot and leg outward and place it on your lap at the top of your thigh. Alternatively you can place one foot on top of the lower calf. Inhale deeply and lengthen your spine drawing your shoulders back allowing the shoulder blades to gently slide closer, relaxing the shoulders. Exhale and allow yourself to be rooted from your pelvic floor gently softening in to the pose. Relax breathing steady and rhythmically.

Nun (The primordial waters/collective unconsciousness)

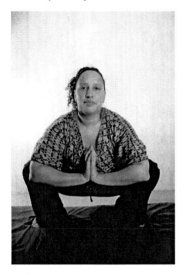

Nun relates to (the mythological) primordial waters or (the cosmic) boundless universe, which is the macrocosm of the womb in the physical realm. This is why Sanuy-nun is seen when Afrikan women give birth. Sanuy~nun is perfect for women in pregnancy. Afrikan women have been giving birth in this position for thousands of years.

This tends to be a natural position as gravity allows the baby to easily be born where a lying on your back with your legs up goes against gravity. This is a Greek invention used today in hospitals it creates struggle, distress and bonding disruption. In the position of Nun especially in the last weeks of pregnancy to latter part of the 3rd trimester this position assists the baby to move into the correct position for labour. If the baby is in a breech position or you have cervical suture do not perform Sanuy~nun and also if you are enduring painful haemerroids and varicose veins.

Begin by standing and place palms together in taful in front of your chest bring the body down into a squat position keeping the back straight.

Keep your knees bending over your toes and use your elbows to open your Knees and stretch out the pelvis and hips. Straighten your spine as much as you can as you will be leaning forward. Hold comfortably for 9 breaths.

The benefits of sanuy - nun are:

1. The stretching of the pelvic region and raising a healthy blood supply to this region through the breath
2. Increase circulation
3. Release premenstrual tension
4. Helps to release tension ease aches and pains
5. Boost fertility
6. Tones the inner thigh and abdominals
7. Strengthens the knees, bones and ligaments in the legs
8. Develops balance

In Sanuynun you can also perform *Hikau* (mantra) YAANUN 46 times for vitality

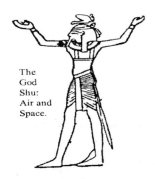

The God Shu: Air and Space.

SHU Pa Raafur Istamzaab "The Raising Position"

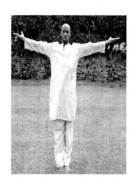 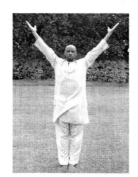 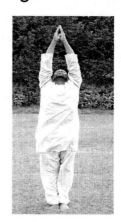

SHU, often called the 'complete breathing technique' by some Yogis. For Complete Breath the arms are raised slowly sideways and upwards during breath retention of this exercise the arms should be overhead.

When performing the complete breath the diaphragm undergoes expansion allowing for brief dislodgement of internal abdominal organs to experience a massage and to gently be relocated during exhalation.

The breathing technique that improves the co-ordination of several systems of the body is both the Complete Breathing technique, which incorporates all three, diaphragm, intercostals and clavicle breathing. This is where the expansion of the diaphragm, ribs, sternum and lungs come into play by steady slow and continuous inhalation of air through the nose and an equal exhalation occurs to expel the air with the sound YAASHUUUUUUU.

SHU also adds to the legs, calves and toe muscles by toning them as you rise on your toes. Shu develops your sense of balance and self trust.

Use hikau Yaa Shu 38 times to draw the healing forces of sekhem throughout your being through each breath.

Earth
Katuf~ Bagum: Shoulder Stand or
"Pa Banur": The Candle.

Katuf Bagum or Candle will have a wonderful effect on the body as it stimulates the thyroid and opens the sekhemic flow of energy in the internal organs via the lay lines of the body known as meridians.

Begin by lying on your back in supine position, hands at the sides of the body, palms on the floor. Bring the chin in towards the chest, which assist the movement. The spinal column must be flat as possible.

If beginners are unable to keep they're backs flat they may start with their knees bent. The legs are raised slowly and together in one continuous movement with grace and deliberateness until they reach a vertical position.

Begin to raise the buttocks and push the legs up vertically and raising the entire torso up balancing on the shoulders supporting your back with your hands. Keep your hands on your back by the kidneys with your fingers turning towards the spinal centre, adjust as you see fit align the body focusing on perfection and the straightness of a candle. Bring the elbows in and slightly more close together.

The benefits of Katuf Bagum are:
1. Stimulates the thyroid gland
2. Stretches the spinal column
3. Massages heart, lungs
4. Encourages good circulation of the blood
5. Prevents sluggishness
6. Assist in the relief of depression and poor sleeping patterns
7. Opens the flow of sekhemic energy in the internal organs, kidneys, small stomach, and gall bladder.

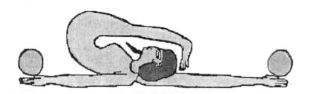

Geb: The Plough

This Sanuy is powerful as it works the entire spine, which contains the spinal cord, influencing the sympathetic nervous system.

The thyroid gland also benefits from Geb with an increase of fresh blood supply, flowing to the area of the neck, throat and head.

This gland controls the metabolism and stimulates the youthfulness of the body. When not functioning at its optimum level the body's skin, becomes wrinkled and dry, blood pressure is low, sexual activity decreases with physical and mental laziness in tow.

The thyroid is the gland most likely to cause overweight and underweight in people, has under-activity of this gland cause the release of hormones to be insufficient which impedes physical and mental growth in children. Over-activity of the thyroid gland shows the exact opposite which cause increase in height, overweight, excitable and nervous.

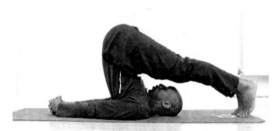

In adults the over activity of the gland may cause some of the same conditions he/she may lose weight and become irritable with a rapid pulse rate, eyes also tend to bulge and glaze

Begin by lying on your back in supine position, hands at the sides of the body, palms on the floor. Bring the chin in towards the chest, which assist the movement. The spinal column must be flat as possible.

If beginners are unable to keep they're backs flat they may start with their knees bent. The legs are raised slowly and together in one continous movement with grace and deliberatness until they reach a vertical position.

Begin to raise the buttocks and push the legs up vertically and raising the entire torso up balancing on the shoulders supporting your back with your hands. Now you are in the candle position lower your legs over and away from your head. Allow the toes to touch the floor. Deepening the stretch, and point the toes in towards the head. If your feet do not touch the floor at first, with practise your

spine will lenghthen and your weight will eventual bear down. Always be relaxed and patient allow for no jerky movements as the practice of smai is graceful in all its aspects and any jerks will be detrimental to your well being. This completes the stretch acting on all regions of the vertebrae. Raise the legs and back into Pa Banur the candle and slowly bend the knees toward the head, place the hands on the mat palms facing down and unravel the spine dropping the body and legs towards the floor back into a supine position. Keep the back of the head firmly on the ground again avoiding any jerky movements.
Lie in mummy and relax.

The benefits of this sanuy include:
Physically
1. Brings balance to the thyroid
2. Calms the nerves and is very reviving and is useful for tiredness
3. Send fresh blood flow towards the head, the brain and the face hence preventing wrinkles and lines
4. This movement is beneficial to the spleen and the sexual glands
5. The Sanuy Geb also stimulates the liver, assisting decongestion and cleansing, massaging the pancreas and kidneys
6. Useful for diabetics due to its effect on the pancreas
7. Works against constipation
8. Is effective against cellututis and obesity by improving the function of the colon

Mentally
1. Enhances good posture and inner balance
2. Relieves insomnia and restless sleep.

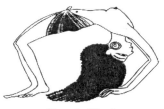
Kemetic Wheel

Shen: The Wheel
Begin in the supine position of lying on your back, legs outstretched palms by your side facing up. Bend your Knees and bring your heels towards your buttocks keep your feet hip-width apart and flat on the floor. Bend the arms backwards and place your palms just above the shoulders with the fingers directed towards your feet.
Inhale Raise your pelvis and hips upwards then press your fingers into the floor and push upwards keeping your feet rooted to the floor. Your shoulder blades will draw inwards and into your back allow this as long as the shoulders do not

tighten up. If the shoulders do tighten widen them a bit by bringing the arms out.

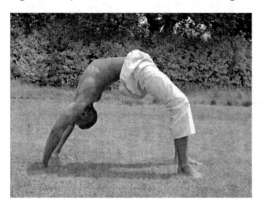

Spread your fingers and push further into an arch forming the SHEN hold for several breaths. Bend the elbow and draw the head in towards the chest while lowering yourself onto your back and exiting the Sanuy.

The benefits of this sanuy include:
Physically
1. The entire spine maintaining it's strength and suppleness
2. The strengthening of the thighs and hips
3. The wrists, forearms, shoulders and spine all receive a stretch
4. Opens up the chest cavity increasing the lung capacity.
5. The movement also strengthens and tones the buttocks, legs, chest, back shoulders and wrists
6. Stimulates the lymph, reproductive and digestive systems
7. Assist in the infertility, osteoporosis, back-ache and asthma
8. Stimulate the thyroid and pituitary gland
9. Helps to increase your stamina

Mentally
1. Energises the mind
2. Relieves mild depression
3. Relieves anxiety and reduces stress

Do not do this movment if you have high or low blood pressure, back, knee or neck injury or carpol tunnel syndrome.

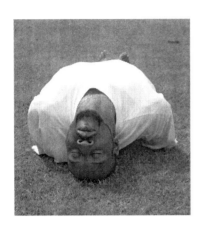

Manjet 'The Boat of Re'

The manjet is like a semi inverted Sanuy it entails more of a backward bend and is viewed as a counter pose to the Katuf Bagum Sanuy alongside the Shen Sanuy.

Begin by laying flat on your back and place your palms under your thighs and turn the palms upwards, breathing gently and regularly. Keep the legs straight and point the toes upwards and the heel down in to the floor. Raise your body upwards turning the shoulder blades in and pressing down on to the elbows as the upper body is raised of the ground. The legs remain on straight and on the ground. Balance your weight on your elbows, arch the back and drop your head backwards lowering the body on top of the head. It is important that you keep the weight on the elbows as your head only touches the ground slightly. Now breathe a little more deeply but maintain a regular breath. Allow the chest to open up further and keep the shoulder blades together. You may gaze directly behind you on a certain spot or object if you need to focus.

When finished press down on the elbows and lift the head of the ground and back into a tilt position before lowering the head. Now just allow the body to drop gently back down on to the mat in mummy Sanuy.

The benefits of this Sanuy include:
1. The stretching of the intestines and abdominals.
2. It promotes deep breathing and assist in the alleviation of backache.
3. The pelvis is also stretched
4. The shoulders and arms are strengthened and toned.
5. The Thyroid, thymus and pineal glands are stimulated.
Focus is the solar plexus.

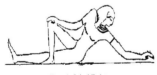

Kemetic Spinal Twist

Geb/Spinal Twist

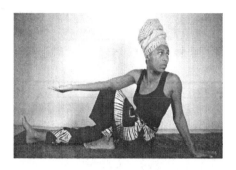

This sanuy is another wonderful posture that works the entire spine.

Begin by sitting on the mat legs outstretched in front of you, feet together. Bend or double up the right leg and bring your feet alongside your left knee, let the anklebone touch the outside of the knee. The right foot is flat on the ground and parallel with the left leg. Now place the right arm back and lean back slightly (only a touch) with the right hand flat on the floor fingers spread wide a part. Allow the hand to take your weight. Now draw your body up towards your thigh, as your back should be upright as much as possible. Now place your left arm across your torso and lever it around to the right knee making it parallel with the outstretched left leg. Now with this outstretched arm, turn the palm facing upwards.

The left arm is inducing the shoulders to turn and therefore creating the twist in the spine without offering any resistance. The head now turns looking over the right shoulder at the same time stretching the neck completing 'Geb spinal twist'. Hold for 9 breaths.

The Sanuy is also practised on the other leg where the left leg is bent and the left arm and hand is placed on the floor etc.

Concentrate on the relaxation of the spinal structure and the shoulders and follow mentally the twist from the sacrum up to the skull.

The benefits of this sanuy include:
1. Stretches and lengthens the spine and all the muscles and ligaments in the spinal vertebrae.
2. Tones up the muscles in the back through the rush of blood flow.
3. Tone up the entire organism of the body as it works the nerves of the spinal chord
4. Stimulate and has a great effect on the nervous system commonly called the immune system which is strengthened by the spinal twist
5. Increases the flexibility of the spine
6. Removes and relieves muscular problems in the back
7. Massages the abdominals
8. Positive effects on the spleen, gall bladder, kidneys, liver and bowls
9. Develops the sekhemic energy
10. Promotes peace of mind and stability.

Sitting Nut/Forward Bend

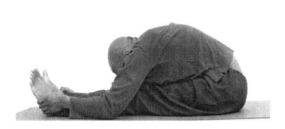

Sit with legs extended. Inhale and press your hands down into the floor to lengthen your spine, bring your lower back in and upward making the back tall.

Inhale and bring your arms over head. Exhale, bend forward and grasp your toes or alternatively grasp your big toes with your index and middle fingers.

Inhale and extend your belly up through the top of your head. Tilt your pelvis forward and draw your lower back in anchor your thighs down and exhale widening your elbows out and draw your torso forward towards your feet. Keep the legs engaged and straight. Bend the waist like a hinge and lead with the heart, bring the head forward moving towards the feet.

Repeat this stretch 3 times and hold each time for 9 breaths 19 for the more advance.

The benefits of this sanuy include:
1. Stretches the spine, hamstring and calves,
2. Improves digestion
3. Stimulates the lymph and reproductive systems,
4. Helps relieve menstrual and menopause discomfort,
5. Improves liver, kidney and colon function
6. Massages the abdominal organs.
7. Increases elasticity in the joints.
8. Alleviates high blood pressure and infertility.
9. Keeps you youthful.
10. Reduces fatigue and insomnia
11. Soothes the nervous system
12. Relieves stress, anxiety and mild depression
13. Develops concentration and sekhem energy
14. Assists in meditation.

Contra-indication
Lower back injury asthma
Pregnancy (use variations)

Mental Transformation Sanuyaats

Selket Scorpion

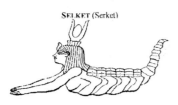

SELKET (Serket)

The movement of the legs in Selket utilises the muscles of the entire lower back and the muscles of the lower back is strengthened

The practitioner lays flat on their stomach with the forehead place down on to the mat. The legs are close together (at a beginners level) the hands are made into a fist and tucked under the thighs. Alternatively the hands and arms are stretched out forward and above the head, or place palms facing down just under the thighs.

It is very important that all advance and beginners start by using what is termed half scorpion where one leg is raised on inhale; raise the leg as far as it can go keeping the leg straight, and hold; lower the leg on the exhale.

Relax by turning the head onto it side. Repeat the movement on the opposing leg. Then raise both legs together using the same process of inhaling and lowering on exhale. The length of time you hold the breath can vary between 3 breaths up to 9 breaths, however, it is important not to exceed 9 breaths.

The benefits of this sanuy include:

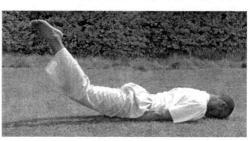

1. Utilises the muscles of the entire lower back
2. The muscles of the lower back are strengthened considerably
3. Increases the flexibility of the back
4. Tones the lumber and sacral region and is quite simple so anyone can perform it
5. Works and stimulates the kidneys
6. Stimulates the nervous system
7. Stimulates the solar plexus.

Wadjet/UREAUS Cobra

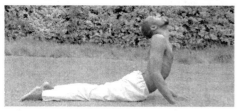

In supine position place hands palms down just under your shoulders. Keep the elbows on the ground and close to your sides. Turn the toes in and inhale. Raise the chest off the floor pushing upwards using your hands and spreading your fingers whilst arching the torso up in the slow graceful movement of the cobra. Concentrate on the third eye and turn your toes out. Inhale and Exhale holding as long as possible, keeping the shoulders relaxed. Repeat for as long as possible.

The benefits of this sanuy include:
Physically
1. Massages the muscles in the back
2. Increases the spine flexibility
3. Expands the rib cage
4. Brings relief from asthma
5. Gently massages internal organs
6. Assist in the relief of numerous menstrual problems

Mentally
1. Develops the faculty of concentration
2. Releases sekhem energy helping you to realise your full potential

Sebek Crocodile

Start n a Dub/Scarab child position place both arms in front of you on the floor keeping them wide and bent at the elbows making the form of a KA.

Draw the left leg back keeping the right knee bent.

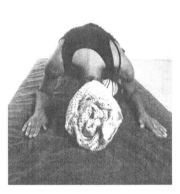 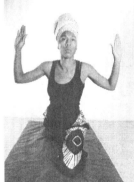

Remain sitting slightly on your heel and inhale and raise your head and chest and arms of the floor stretching and arching the spine. Once you are balanced exhale and gently settle back down to the floor keeping the arms in the same position of a KA.

Draw the left leg back into a kneeling position of the Scarab. Repeat drawing the right leg back.

Benefits of this sanuy include:
1. Stretches the hips, thighs
2. Stretches the spine
3. Opens the chest
4. Develops flexibility in the hips and back
5. Strengthens toes and ankle

FIRE
Pa Bast/ the Cat

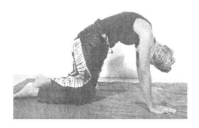 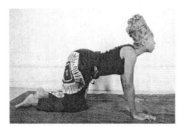

This Sanuy opens the back and stretches the spine and is beneficial for menstrual problems delivering a flow of blood to the nervous system through the spine. Begin on all fours with your hands in line with your shoulders and your knees and legs parallel but slightly apart. Inhale and raise the entire back arched upwards into a hump stretching the shoulder blades and bending the head inwards resting the chin on the collar - bone looking toward the chest. Exhale and slowly lift the head and at the same time drop the abdominals down towards the mat and curve the back inwards.

The benefits of this sanuy include:
1. Increase flexibility of the spine
2. Strenghens and tones the abdominal region
3. Increases the strength in shoulders, arms, wrists and thghs
4. Increases circulation
5. Improves digestion

Approaching the Higher Self

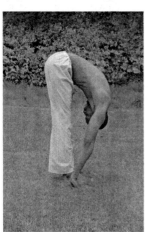

Standing Nut/Forward Bend
Begin by standing with your feet parallel, spread your toes and root yourself right down through all four corners of your feet. Inhale and raise you're your arms out to the side or push the arms up from the centre of your body extending your lower torso pushing up through your finger tips and maintain the length.
Exhale and bend forward reaching for your toes or the floor. Hold for a few breaths.

Benefits of this sanuy include:
Physically
1. Lengthens spine
2. Developing suppleness and elasticity
3. Mobilize joints
4. Rejuvenate the nervous system
5. Stretches hamstrings and muscles of the back of the leg
6. Increases blood supply to the brain
7. Burns of calories

Mentally
1. Gentle enhances concentration
2. Dissolves laziness
3. Stimulating intelligent capacities

Heru/Haru

Heru/Haru sanuy in the Indian system of yoga is called the mountain posture this is interesting as Har means "on high".

Begin by standing with feet slightly apart and shoulders relaxed and hands down by your sides turning your palms facing forwards. Feel your weight evenly distributed on both feet and root yourself in the ground. Raise your head up so the neck and spine is stretched upward as if pulled by a thin thread. Lift you chest and breathe deeply and evenly pushing out the stomach on the inhale and bringing the stomach back towards the spine on the exhale. Listen to the sound of your breath and continue up to 9 times. There should be no tension in you
The meditation is on Heru who has conquered the lower natures.

Benefits of this sanuy include:
Physically
1. Aligns the body posture
2. Assist in the distribution of weight evenly in the body.
3. Improves balance

Mentally
1. Relieves mental tension
2. Promotes calm and self-assurance

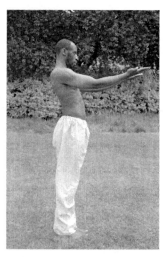

Henu (Anpu, Heru, Set)
Standing Position
From Heru you move in to Anpu also known as Anubis. This sanuy is known as a warrior pose and used in the form of tension dynamics.

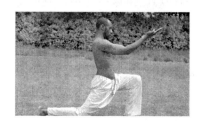

Begin by standing in Heru then bend the elbow at a 45 degree angle raise both hands up directly in front of you palms facing upwards fingers together and thumbs in. Then draw the left leg back bending the knee and lowering it to the ground (advance students don't touch the floor), Bring the arm of the bended leg across to the right shoulder curling the hand in to a fist and bring the outstretched arm around to the side of the shoulder circulating the forearm and bending the elbow palm facing forward hold for 4 breaths and increase to 9 breaths.
Repeat on the otherside of the body.

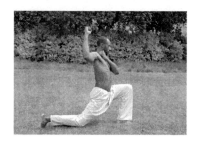

The benefits of this sanuy include:
Physically
1. Promotes strength legs
2. Develops flexibility in the legs
3. Increase flexibility in the thighs, abdomen, and back
4. Increases flexibility in the foot and toes
5. Increase strength in the buttocks, feet and ankles
6. Promotes and increase balance, posture in the back, legs and spine.
7. Opens the hips and groin area
8. Opens the chest and strengthens the shoulders
9. Increases mobility in the shoulder blades.
10. Increase circulation in the organs and tones the abdominals.
Mentally
1. Eliminates lethargy and laziness
2. Promotes strength of mind
3. Develops courage and fearlessness
4. Imparts resilience and strength

Maat

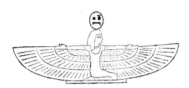

This sanuy seems simple yet it requires a high level of concentration and balance.

Stand with your feet shoulder widths apart; raise both arms from the sides laterally away from the body, keeping the fingers together stretching and pointing. Then turn the head to the right, followed by the feet keeping the rest of the body facing forward to give a gentle twist in the spine, bend the back foot going down on your knee and lean back and sit on your back heel. Maintain the stretch in the arms keeping them up, straight and level with your shoulders. Sit and breathe for 3 deep breaths.

Rise up and reverse each movement, by turning the feet pointing forwards, then the head and lastly drop the arms down to the sides. Repeat the process by turning the head and the feet to the left.

The benefits of this sanuy include:
Physically
1. Invigorates the circulation
2. Strengthens the shoulders
3. Increases flexibility in the chest and shoulders
4. Stretches the thighs and knees
5. Increase stamina

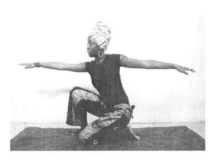

Mentally
1. Develops determination, single-mindedness
2. Improves mental concentration and physical balance
3. Reduces mental stress
4. Alleviates anxiety

Maat helps the body to feel lighter and increases sekhemic flow to the lungs and heart.

Aset

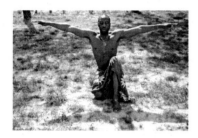

Stand with feet slightly apart and inhale raise both arms laterally take a step back with the left leg and bend the left knee going down on the knee and lean back sitting on the heel keeping the back straight and the arms raised

Benefits of this sanuy include:
1. Strengthens shoulders and upper back
2. Strengthens thighs
3. Tones the abdominals
4. Opens the chest
5. Strengthens the ankles and toes
6. Develops balance

Contraindications
Ankle and knee injuries

Aset Embrace

Stand legs shoulder width apart and bring the arms out towards the sides, away from the body stretching the chest and keeping the palms facing each other.

This is can be a graceful movement with the use of the breath or this can be used as a form of dynamics or tension by tensing the arms has you bring the palms to face each other in front of the torso contracting the muscles of the back and releasing and relaxing the arms moving lightly back to a wide arm stretch. Inhale as the arms are wide and slowly exhale as the arms move forward and hands face moves downward and towards each other tensing or resisting.

Benefits of this sanuy include:
Physically
1. Improves circulation
2. Develops and stimulates the lungs
3. Strengthens the nervous system

Mentally
1. Promotes calm
2. Relieves stress and anxiety

Sekhemic
Strengthens the auric field

increases eletro-magnetic energy
Increases sekhem energy
Rejuvenates sekhemic energy throughout the entire body

Djed Asaru

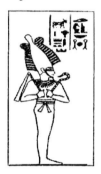

Begin by standing very straight crossing the arms over your chest right arm over the left fingers on the collar bone. Close the eyes and concentrate on the spine. Gently push out the stomach and inhale for a count of 4 and hold the breath for a count of 2 exhale slowly through the nose for a count of 4 pulling the abdominals in and rest for 2 counts. Keep the cycles of rhythmic breathing going in Djed Asaru as this position is a meditative state. With the arms crossed over the chest creates a pyramid and is useful for the Heper (heart) and Ab (solar plexus) chakra and for regenerative purposes. This pose can be used also to induce a deep, a restful and cell stimulating sleep.

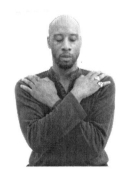

The benefits of this sanuy include:
Physically
1. Rejuvenates the heart
2. Rejuvenates and stimulates the solar plexus
Mentally
1. Increase blalance
2. Promotes concentration

Also see Haru

Establishment Sanuyaat

Rus~Baqum Headstand

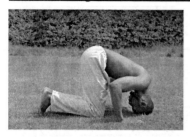 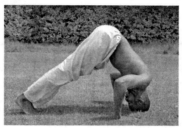 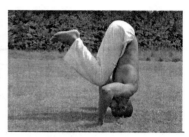

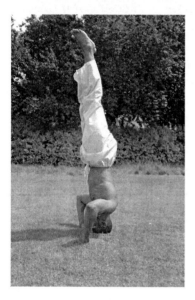

This advance Sanuy is highly recommended for its development of concentration and the stimulation of the pineal gland the melanin factory in your brain.

Begin by kneeling position Heru sitting, place your arms on the mat and form and Aset Taruh/lock widening your elbows so that you form a triangle shape with your forearms and hands which are locked together via the fingers. Place your head inside the hands, rolling it so the back of your head is up against the inside of your fingers and you are resting on the top of your head. Raise your body by stretching out your legs behind you and roll forward so you are now on top of your head. The alternative is to create a triangle with the hands and head.The head being at the top of the triangle.

Now Inhale and walk your feet towards your elbows. Exhale and raise your feet of the ground bending at the knee and pushing the feet straight upwards concentrate on perfection. Hold for 9-45 breaths Inhale/exhale come down keeping your head on the ground and back to kneeling position. Then turn and lay on your back to let the blood naturally flow back to normal for a few moments

The benefits of this sanuy include:
Physically
1. Strenghthens the respiratory system
2. Increases circulation
3. Rest the heart through gravity (returns the venous blood flow towards the heart)
4. Slowing down the rate of the heart beat and breathing

5. Rejuvenates the entire body

Mentally
1. Increases memory
2. Increases concentration
3. Stimulates intellectual capacity
4. Promotes the sensory capacities

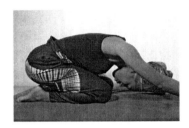

Khepri/ Dub/scarab

Sit on your heels with your shoulders nice and even. Bow forward and gently place your torso and upper body on your thighs, bring your arms forward and lengthen the arm reaching forward. Stretch the sides of your body from your hips to your shoulders.

Now allow the arms to go limp and relax palms facing down.

As an option you may draw the arms back towards your feet and let the shoulders widen turn the palms upward alongside your feet.

Benefits of this sanuy include:

Physically
1. Alleviates the head, neck and chest
2. Opens the pelvis hips and lower back
3. Stretches the ankles knees and hips
4. Opens up the upperback relieving tension in the shoulder

Mentally
1. Calms the mind
2. Reduces stress and lessens fatigue

Do not do this if you have an ankle, knee or hip injury

If pregnant keep the knees apart and do not put too much pressure on your abdominals a cushion or thick layers of blankets can be used between the abdominal region and thighs for support.

Asar/Karast (Mummy)

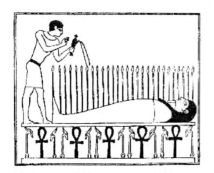

Lie flat on your back, eyes closed, legs slightly apart, and hands by your sides, palms facing upwards. Stay in this position for a minute or two. Concentrate on the breath. Take a long slow inhalation inviting the breath into your lungs and filling the upper body by applying mid and lower breathing. Hold the breath for a count of 3; as you count pull the sekhem in to every cell of your being. Exhale with complete control nice and slow. Continue with this line of breathing upto 9 breaths expanding the ribs cage and pushing the stomach up towards the ceiling. You can continue to breathe deeply but as normally as you can for a complete 10 min. This sanuy intergrates the benfits of your yoga practise and allows the body to gather energy. The focus is to nurture and centring yourself. You do this so that you may continue to nurture others in the world, sharing your peace, tranquillity and calm.

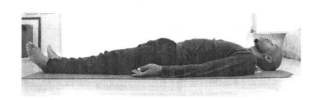

Benefits of the sanuy include:
Physically
1. Increases lung capacity
2. Increases internal muscle control
3. oxygeneates the blood
4. Alchalis the body
5. Detoxifies the body
6. Lowers blood pressure
7. Reduces fatigue
8. Triggers relaxation throughout the entire nervous system

Mentally
1. Calms the mind
2. Promotes tranquillity and ease
3. Produces a feeling of being nurtured
4. Rejuvenates the mind

Nefertum

The session is completed with a meditation sitting in Nefertum pose.

This can last between 10 min to a full hour. (Please refer to meditation poses and meditation exercises)

18 minute Morning set

1. SHU
Stand erect and extend arms out raise the arms overhead with thumbs touching inhaling deeply as you raise arms and rise on to your toes.
Exhale YAA SHU slowly has you drop arms and back onto your feet.

Repeat 9x slowly increase to 36x 2 minutes

2. NUT
Raise arms overhead thumbs touching and arch backwards and exhale, slowly bend forward to touch toes.
Repeat 9x slowly increase to 36x 2 minutes
THESE 2 COMBINED CHARGES ELECTRO-MAGNETIC FIELD

3. WIDE LEG STRETCH
Sit spread legs wide apart. Now forward bend to the centre for a few seconds.
Stretch towards the left foot and lower the head to the left knee, with deep sekhem breath hold for 1 min
End. Inhale pull in stomach squeeze buttocks hold has long as possible and release slowly exhaling.
Relax and repeat stretch on right side. 1 minute

4. SELKET
On stomach, place forehead on the floor, mat or cushion place hands palms down under thighs (beginners use fists)
And inhale as you raise legs straight and high as possible and hold as long as possible. Exhale lowering your legs.
Repeat for 2 min
Relax for 1 min

5. WADJET/Arat
In supine position place hands palms down just under your shoulders.
Keep the elbows on the ground and close to your sides.
Turn the toes in and raise the chest of the floor pushing upwards using your hands spread your fingers. Arching the torso up in cobra concentrate on the third eye and turn your toes out. Inhale and Exhale holding as long as possible keep the shoulders relaxed.

Repeating as long as possible.
Continue for 3 min
Relax for 1 min

6. GEB The Plough

In supine position raise legs and hips perpendicular to the floor supporting them with your hands and move into Katuf Bagum/Shoulder Stand placing your weight onto your shoulders, neck and upper arms.
Keeping your legs straight gently lower them down to the floor behind and away from the head hold for 30 sec increase to 1 min Inhale and Exhale.
Resting for 1 min

7. Easy Pose/Adept

Sit in Easy pose and lie back your hands folded in Aset lock on the navel.
Meditate at 3rd eye. 2 min
Increase according to your leisure.

This set raises the Sekhem energy and is an excellent preparation for meditation.

Patarugshil-Re...
The Journey of Re

Position 1.
Asaru/mummy
Deep relaxation pose

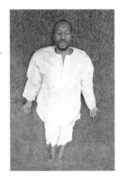

Position 2.
Taful Exhale
Prayer pose the
male and female
energies coming
together balancing

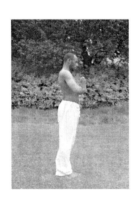

Position 3.
TheDuat/Amenta
Inhale
Backward bend

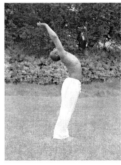

Position 4.
Standing
Nut/sky exhale
Forward bend

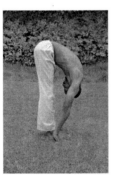

Position 5. Right
leg stretch inhale

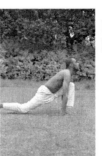

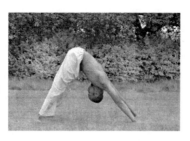

Position 6.
Pyramid exhale

Position 8. Plane
Hold the breath

Position 7.
Arat/Cobra inhale

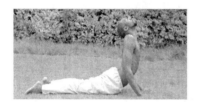

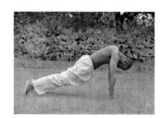

Position 9.
Pyramid exhale

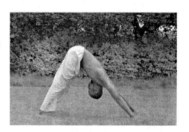

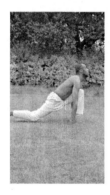

Position 10.
Leg stretch inhale

Position 11. Nut
inhale into
Amenta exhale

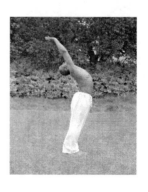

Repeat changing leg.

Patarugshil-Re...
The Journey of Re

Take 3-10 minutes a day
All you need is a space measuring 2 square meters and it cost nothing.
This acts on all the organism of the body and is not limited to one part only.

- *Patarugshil-re* tones up the digestive system by the alternate stretching and compression of the abdominal region, it massages the liver, the spleen, intestines and kidneys activating the digestion and getting rid of constipation and dyspepsia (disorders of the stomach)

- *Patarugshil-re* Strengthens the abdominal muscles, the arms and the wrists.

- *Patarugshil-re* Synchronises movement with breathing, thoroughly ventilating the lungs, oxygenates the blood and acts as a de-toxicant, because it get rid of a large amount of carbon dioxide and other toxic gases through the respiratory tract.

- *Patarugshil-re* Increases cardiac activity and the flow of blood throughout the system, which is ideal for the health of the body.

- *Patarugshil-re* It combats hypertension and palpitations and warms up the extremities.

- *Patarugshil-re* Tones up the nervous system by successfully stretching and bending the spine, it regulates the function of the sympathetic and para-sympathetic systems and helps to promotes sleep.

- *Patarugshil-re* The memory improves.

- *Patarugshil-re* It relieves worry and anxiety.

- *Patarugshil-re* It stimulates and normalizes the activity of the endocrine glands, the thyroid in particular through the movement of the neck.

- *Patarugshil-re* Refreshes the skin and if done correctly there is a slight sweating and moisture may appear. Under African skies a few minutes is enough. The skin will be well irrigated so that it reflects good health and the complexion will clear.

- *Patarugshil-re* Improves the muscle structure throughout the body:

- ***Patarugshil-re*** Neck, shoulders, arms, wrist, back, abdominals as well as the thighs, calves and ankles without inducing hardening of the muscles.

- ***Patarugshil-re*** Potential backache is held at bay are easily held at bay due to the strengthening of the back.

- ***Patarugshil-re*** In women and girls the bust develops normally and becomes firm regaining any lost in elasticity through stimulation of the glands and strengthening the pectoral muscles.

- ***Patarugshil-re*** Controls activity in the uterus and ovaries, suppressing menstrual irregularity with its accompanying pain, and assist in childbirth.

- ***Patarugshil-re*** Increases immunity to disease.

- ***Patarugshil-re*** Provides grace and ease to the movements of the body preparing the body for sports of all kinds.

- ***Patarugshil-re*** Revives and maintain a spirit of youthfulness, producing health and strength and longevity an asset beyond price.

Hand Positions

TAARUH ISTAMZAAB

Hand gestures or positions locks, guides energy flow and reflexes to the brain. By curling, crossing stretching and touching the finger tips to the thumb we can talk to the body and mind as each finger corresponds with the different parts of the body and mind and are interlink with psychic channels.

If you place enough pressure (but not so much that you whiten the finger tips) you will feel the flow of energy through these channels up the arms.

The thumb represents the ego.

Shu Taruh
Index finger
Jupiter
Stimulating
knowledge
Ability
Organ Lungs

Aset Taruh
Middle finger
Saturn
Stimulating
Patience
Nurturing
Organ Liver

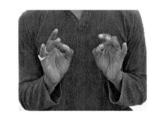

RE Taruh
Ring finger Sun
Stimulating energy
health and intuition
Organ Circulation/Sex

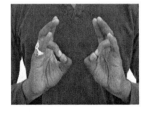

Anubu Taruh
Little finger Mercury
Stimulating clear
intuitive
communication
Organ Heart

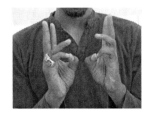

Aset lock/grip

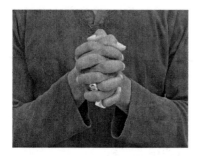

Interlace fingers with left little finger on the bottom and right index finger on top for men and the left for women. The Aset mounds at the base of the thumbs are pressed together channelling sensuality, sexuality and glandular balance helping to focus and concentrate.

Taful Taruh

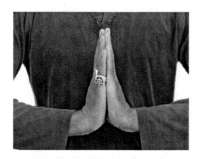

The Prayer pose this is where both palms are pressed together, neutralizing and balancing both male and female principles for cantering.

Ptah Taruh

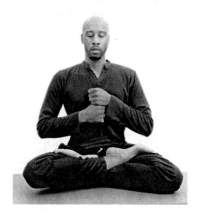

Both hands are curled into a fist the left on the bottom and the right position on the top over and against the solar plexus/sternum for stability balance and centering.

Finger	planet	zodiac	Supreme being/kosmic energy	body
index	Jupiter	sagittarius	Shu	Lungs/thighs
Middle	Saturn	Capricorn	Aset	Liver/bones/knees
Ring	Sun	Leo	Re/Het-Heru	Circulation/sex
little	Mercury	Virgo/Gemini	Anubu	Heart

Chant & Hand gestures

Sound   AH MUN RE TA

Ah: touch index finger to thumb (index =Shu stimulating knowledge and ability.)

Mun: touch middle finger to thumb (middle = Aset patience and giving patience)

Re: touch ring finger to thumb (ring = RE/Hathor giving energy health and intuition)

Ta: little finger to thumb (little = Anubu clear and intuitive communication)

Meditation

"Live in truth, enter silence, there is peace, peace is silence"
The Mind, Scroll 11:53 inscribed by Dr Malachi Z York

The Afrikan Yoga, Hudu and Hanuaat/exercises are meditation through movement and this form of meditation is very useful for the active, rapid mind.

However, meditation through stillness is useful for those who wish to search deeper into the constructs of the soul. This search is to find self and tap into the source of all things, thereby generating internal healing, and mental manifestations of the will on a cosmic etheric and wholistic level.

The smai student/practitioner must be one or you will be many and with many comes confusion not just for you but who ever you come in contact with. You go around and create turmoil and chaos. We are unaware of this so we go about wreaking havoc in people lives thinking we are doing good deeds. This is the mistake of many good doers, leaders, ministers, priests, teachers, and those who claim to be healers. We must be one, centred and balanced or we will walk around with the many in our heads bringing confusion.

Meditation is simply the observation of the mind. The practitioner is being a witness of self, now centering and controlling the mind. (Please refer to The 9 Principles of Tehuti Mental). Meditation is mind control via the self through internal means rather than the numerous forms of mind control via external means. There is much to be said about meditation but rather go through theory; here are a few exercises to experience meditation.

The key thing is to be completely relaxed. Sit in a comfortable position so you can be still for a period of 10 min –1hr

Breathe Meditation

Sit on a chair or on the floor if on the floor you can cross the legs (please refer to Sitting Sanuyaats for Meditation) Pull your spine upwards and make the spine tall. Close the eyes and concentrate on the flow of air entering the nostrils visualise the flow rolling down in to the abdomen filling the torso and pushing the abdomen out, feel the air brush all around your nose and feel it flow out on the exhale allowing the abdomen to deflate, gently pull the abdomen back towards the spine. This movement of breath is the first stage as it slows down and begins to focus the mind on the 'Arush Shiru' nasal chakra this also stimulates the Mer seat in between the eyebrows opening the first eye, the Eye of Horus.

150

The other Arushaats will begin to open do not be concerned for this meditation is simply to observe the breath and by doing so narrowing down the many ramblings of the mind into one gleaming instrument. Oness is the attainment.

The mind will drift and you will be bombarded with many thoughts. Do not worry just gently guide the mind back to the breath and the inhale and exhale of air through the nostrils. With practise the concentration will develop, give yourself time and nurture yourself.

Now Meditiation

The mind has a tendency to live in the future or the past infact most of us are in that state most of the time and therefore unconscious. Unconscious because the past is not real it has gone and you cannot get it back, in the now it does not exist. The future has not happened yet and many of us worry about and project to events that we feel may be of concern or wonderful happenings etc that do not really exist in the now. 'The Now' is real. Meditation assists your conscious awareness of this fact.

Sit on a chair or on the floor keep the spine and head erect just as in the Breath meditation. Close the eyes and concentrate on the flow of breath, entering the nostrils, breath steadily and observe your mind it will begin to wonder either to the past or the future. By observing the minds journey you will be aware of the illusory state. Ask yourself this "Where am I right now". This can also be useful when doing a task and the mind wonders therefore cutting your energy and concentration down to a small percentage, the question becomes "What am I doing right now". The mind will automaticly answer and you will be gently brought back to a state of now. You may have to do this a few times in a session. The Smai student uses this process to be present in any situation.

Candle Meditation

This form of meditation is for concentration, visualization and exercising the First Eye (The Mer Arush). It is also useful for children to develop stillness and focus. Alternatively you can use a small object or a dot on the wall.

Sit using the seated poses for meditation a few few feet away from a candle and focus on the flame. The breath must remain steady and rhythmic. Watch the flame dance and flicker all of your periphery vision will begin to narrow down as you enter into the flame. Slowly narrow the eyes until they naturally close. Keep the image of the flame in the forefront of your mind. This forefront will be between your eyebrows the seat of the first eye, 'The eye of Heru' (The Mer Arush). Keep this focus for as long as you can and use the breath to allow you to go into yourself using the first eye to look within, you will find a place of no mind. Stillness. Peace.

Suggestions for a Beneficial Practise

Afrikan Yoga =A Free Ka (n) science

An affirmation
"To my mental and physical effort I add potential of my spiritual self, its qualities permeate affairs. Its powers flow through my entire being".

Time and Patience

Time is relevant to ones state of consciousness. What do I mean by that? When one is young and full of energy with apparently very little to do and the concentration span is low, time appears to be long. On the other hand when one is older and mastered the art of concentration through meditation, the energy is retained to achieve much, time appears quicker. Another example is you are in an aerobics class jumping up and down to some pumping sped up music your heart is thumping and your lungs have ballooned to the point where they feel they are going to pop. It's an hour long class and you have only done 10 mins. The next day you attend a yoga class and asked to stretch concentrating on your breath, your muscles and blood. You are asked to nurture yourself and take it easy all the movements are slow and deliberate, yet the class finishes before you are even aware and this is an hour and half class. What appears to be long is actually short because ones state of consciousness has shifted.

So time is down to consciousness the higher the consciousness the shorter the time to the point where time and space cease to exist. This point is known as God-consciousness or tapping into the 7th plane of existence. So there are many time zones that are not based on geographic location but also on varied states of existence and consciousness. Take time in your practise and you find that you move from zone to zone, state to state and that your mentality can accommodate much more as it has expanded. At the same time; time is sped up to the point (The black dot) that time and space cease to exist, one with 'All', here and there at the same time. Einstein and other scientist viewed that the key to time travel is to move at the speed of light this is what you do when your consciousness shifts you become more of a light being, less solid, why because your cells have sped up. This works with the breath, meditation and sanuyaats. The best times for beneficial practise is in the morning before 8am; assisting the awakening of the

152

body and mentally preparing and stimulate the practitioner for the rest of the day. You can also practise during the evening before going to bed, however, make this light and shorter as the stretches you use should in no way be over done as the muscles and the body wants to rest and therefore exersion can cause injury.

It is also advised not to rush your forms or to compete with others at achieving the desired outcomes of postures. Take time and use time, be patient and secure in the knowledge you have gained to date use this book to understand what is happening to the body and mind, use the Neteru to gain benefits of nature and always be good to yourself.

Nutrition

The golden rule is not to be excessive or over indulgent in certain foods and drinks i.e. spicey foods, sugary and salty foods, alcohol and drinks that dehydrate the body. The benefits of adequate nutrition are the general homeostasis of the body, providing health and vitality. The consumption of high amounts of sugar can prove to be lethal. A spoon of white refined sugar can lower the immune system by 70%. Now none of the bodily systems and organs functions separately and independently of each other. So how can we assume that the function of the brain and the psychological and emotions processes will not be adversely affected by a substance that is able to affect the performance of the liver, pancreas, lungs, kidneys, gall bladder, spleen heart and other organs. Think of it this way sugar erodes the teeth one of the hardest substance in the body. The Smai practitioners have found that food affect the sub-conscious mind and of course are aware how food can effect ones physical and mental performance.

Sugar in particular dulls the positive capacity of the spirit in ways you could only imagine. An example for this is when eating a sugary snack before going to bed can result in a dream where you are on the run from someone or something, fighting someone or something or witnessing violent actions. These are ripples in the brain circuitry caused by the overwork of the pancreas and adrenals processing the sugar in your digestive system. When over stressed these organs and glands are likely to sympatheticly produce adrenaline the commonly known chemical substance associated with 'fight or flight'. The sugar stimulates the secretion of adrenaline and you are in a battle during the time of rest.

You are in a state of fear and this can happen any time during the day or night. The divine energy and grace that we travel with is nullified through the intake of particular substances that is termed 'pica' non food. Today in modern times which is another way of saying western we are saturated with man made substances labelled as food.

The smai practitioner learns to curb the urges of working against nature in this manner or suffers the consequence immediately. The smai practitioner understands that fresh vegetables and fruit or the lack of them go an extremely long way in effectively making an impact on their health and the health of their community. No matter what social class or ethnicity fresh food cannot be under valued as a key factor in the health of individuals. Fruit and vegetables carry high amounts of nutrients, vitamins and water in a formula that the body can easily absorb to sustain and maintain homeostasis and cellular function. Fruit and vegetables grown by 'Re' sun light in organic soil is the best sources of body building on the planet. This source is not just for the body, organ and cellular function; it also has an affect on how you think, process information and form human relationships. Amunnubi Roakhptah taught that *"Improper diet is another hindrance to spiritual progress. All foods have distinct energies, just as the physical body is formed from the gross physical portions of the foods that are eaten. So the mind is formed from the more subtle portions. If the food is impure the mind also becomes impure"*.

He goes on to say *"what goes into the human body correlates directly to the efficiency with which the brain functions. Recent studies show that certain red food colourings create hyperactivity in children and that refined sugar can cause emotional instability and this is what most parents are starting their children on"*.

In a Guardian article dated: 11/11/04
A study led by the Harvard school of public health in Boston analysed date from more that 100.000 health professionals over 14 years concluded that a diet of fruits and vegetable led to a modest overall reduction in chronic disease, largely because of the impact on preventing heart disease and strokes the department of health has said increasing fruit and vegetable consumption is the most important anti-cancer measure after stopping people smoking.

Green leafy vegetables were strongly associated in a US research study with lowering the risk of cardiovascular disease. Those participating ate at least 5 serving of fruits and vegetables daily had a lower risk (28%) of vascular disease than participants eating fewer that 1.5 potions a day, probably due to the higher intake of nutrients which were not destroyed through cooking. I have found from personal experience that when I take fresh fruit and green leafy vegetables eaten raw I am vibrant, have more energy, mentally sharper and far more sensitive to my surroundings and I have seen similar potency in others with the same eating habits.

Drink Water

Water is ultimately a purifying detoxifying chemical. We are in fact more water beings than earthlings. Our bodies are 70%, 75% water some say more than that and each part of our body right down to the cellular level needs water.

Drinking plenty of water flushes out toxins and baths internal organs. The oxygen regenerates and assists the body's absorption of food, improving the digestive system and the other systems of the body.

Water carries electricity, electro neuro impulses are the fundemental premise of the nervous system. The entire human nervous system consists of these electro neuro impulses carrying messages to and from the brain. This functions well with correct amount of plain water. Drink 6-8 glasses per day to maintain the body's natural equilibrium.

Deep Breathing

A human can do without food for well over a week and up to a month, a human can do without water for days, yet a human is unable to function without air for only a few minutes. This is the magnanimous importance of breath.

The majority of western society practise improper breathing which causes respiratory problems and disease of the body. Breathing from the chest (Tat shallow breathing) and insufficient use of the diaphragm are the main components of western breathing practises.

The smai yogi uses **Deep Breathing** using their whole diaphragm.
Deep Breathing improves bronchial function providing good healthy lung tissue through the proper use of all portions of the lungs preventing colds. Deep breathing improves the quality of the blood. The proper oxygenation of the blood is vital for adequate body function and the immune system. As the overall body organ and every part is dependent upon blood for nourishment. Proper breathing gently massages the internal organs stimulating their actions and encouraging normal functions. The diaphragm is nature's principal instrument for this internal exercise. Deep breathing gives you greater control of your body, increasing circulatory system, develops your mental capabilities and promotes the spiritual side of your nature. Lastly deep breathing simply reduces stress.

Rest and Relaxation

Rest is an important aspect of life as in the principle of rhythm one cannot be on the go all the time and you will have to stop. For many in the city this stopping tends to be against ones own will in the form of sickness and disease.

To avoid this we must return to the laws of Nature (Neteru) meaning to apply relaxation as apart of your way of life, to relax physically and mentally and not just in front of the telly (television). Relaxation is described as the absence of

155

tension, or the absence of muscular contraction. Tension is tightness or a stressed state. Tension is mental thoughts translated into action.

When relaxing the smai student should not imagine climbing a mountain has thought are translated into physical action and you will utilize mountaineering muscles by generating increase contraction to those particular muscles through thought thereby defeating the aim of relaxation. It is easier to relax during exhalation than during inhalation as exhalation takes place during the relaxation of the large diaphragm muscle. When the diaphragm muscle is relaxed the whole body tend to relax and let go of its tension. This exhalation is a release of all tension generally. AS we exhale we should relax more each time as this occurs relaxation becomes more progressive and deepened. One never actually arrives to a complete state or to make the statement in thought 'I am completely relaxed I can go no further' this would mean that one stops making progress and to stop one would have to present conflict to that progress causing tension and muscular spasm. Imagination plays a very large part in relaxation by shaping images and making suggestions to the subconscious mind. The subconscious mind absorbs these subtle intentions of relaxation and implements them. By creating sensory images of the body becoming relaxed, the body will automatically become relaxed. When relaxing the sensation of lightness and weightlessness follows the sensation of extreme heaviness. There are those who can only relax after a stretch, that is to say that stretching actually permits the muscles to relax and weeds out any further tension.

Sleep

According to natures (Neteru) laws we need a certain amount of relaxation unfortunately for many of us this only comes in the form of sleep. Sleep is a wonderful mechanism of nature which western man still will try to defy for the sake of pleasure and recreation. The masters of relaxation tend to be children. Children have so much vigour, life and energy however, when it is time to relax or sleep see how fast they can lock of all activities and allow them selves to go into such a deep sleep they can be carried over rough terrain and not wake up until they are satisfied. See how utterly limp they become and how they sink into the couch, chair or bed leaving an imprint, it is best to take a leaf out of their book in the art of relaxation. The thorough rest allows them to be completely within them selves and gives them the power to be so full of energy.

There are adults who also have the ability to relax completely they tend to be calm and serene not allowing agitating thoughts to take them into deepened states of worry and anxiety. The most successful business people have this tendency has they take the time to rest from work or power nap (snooze) during working hours, rejuvenating themselves to work in jovial non-irritated manner.

Sleep for an adult is around 8 hours (horus) and for a child it is close to 12 hours.

This is so the body can rejuvenate and cells replenish without the destruction we put it through while we are awake or in action.

This period of sleep is recommended to be the one of the most nourishing on earth and even more so if it is done in complete darkness between 10pm and 6am. The darkened state is important as any form of external light such as light from a street lamp or bathroom or hall lamp in the case of children or even the little red light that is often beaming from some electric item in your bedroom can effect the rich flow of melatonin from the pineal gland.

The smai student does not really sleep the smai practitioner rests and regenerate. A technique used to maintain youth and vigour in the city through sleep is to take a black sheet and cover your bedroom window, all electricity must be switched off and the room must be pitched in complete darkness.

To go further one may sleep on your back arms crossed over your chest right over left in the form of Asar (Osiris) thereby creating a pyramid. Science has already proven that organic objects placed within a pyramid structure decays far slower.

Positive Affirmations
Affirmation = A FIRM(ing) ATION (action-doing).
Firming one self- self-belief to self-knowing.
Affirmation is the stabilising transference of self in a context through word sound

"As a man thinks in his heart so is he" (or so he becomes)
Our beliefs systems do determine to an extent how our lives are run.
A positive attitude will produce positive results in our lives.
Our thoughts are the calayst of our creations on a physical level.
They form our abundance or our lack, our achievements and our failures. Thoughts have weight, shape, form and colour.
That is why positive affirmations thought (intent) and word sound is so relevant to balanced health. Unknowingly we say affirmations everyday when we put ourselves down phases such as "I don't think I can do that" or "I'm not good enough" some have gone far enough to say "I'm ugly", well guess what, eh that is exactly what you become. Our very cells and genes can be transformed with thought being the only instrument.

Positive uses of Affirmations
An affirmation is used to help you achieve your goals and the key element is to place your self in the now when you use your affirmation.

"I must become a better businessman" or "I will become a better businessman", still keeo you outside the door not crossing the threshold of change and transformation. You are still treading a mill and back to square one.

"I am a better businessman" takes one immediately across the threshold.

The intent of the affirmation is a crucial element; any space for doubt will throw the effect of a postive affirmation off, confusing the mind and body. Affirmations are said after a meditation or smai session/practise when one has been centralised by these particular activities. The key is to be in a balanced state so that the conscious and unconscious mind works together in harmony. Remember whatever you send out to mother father universe in thought the Kosmos universe sends back to you.

Epilogue

Remember Mastery is not being picture perfect and therefore incapable of surrendering one self to the desires of mortals. That means has a master you still can find your self in powerless situations and are able to sulk, get angry or even scoff at others. No. Mastery is not the inabilitiy to fall or trip. Mastery is being able to transform and transcend the challenges of irritation frustration and self-rightousness as they inevitable will appear. Mastery is acknowledging your capabilities and working those abilities to their full capacity to reach the next level Once mastery is achieved there is a point of being. Just being and this being can come at any point in your life beyond your life situation. Primarily it must be understood that you have the power right now to achieve this point. Now being the operative word not when you go to a class or wait for the next teacher to come along it must be understood that you and your life situations are that teacher. You and your life situations are the initiation and the journey to Being. On this journey you no doubt will come across pain, suffering, internal turmoil, confusion due to the lack of self-awareness, ego and the laws of vibration, polarity, gender etc. Yet this is also a marvellous time has it gives you the opportunity to let go. See the hopelessness and emptyiness of the life filled with ego, desire and hankering. Once you want to change this in your life then and only then are you are ready for Smai/Yoga as you are ready to die and be reborn by experiencing the flip side to the negativity. The master chooses to experience joy, abundance, love, peace, beauty, one-ness and clarity, because this is the true reality of life, utilising the very same divine principles.

There are ones who have arrived at the title master, teacher or leader and even people in general who seek to manipulate other human beings, environment etc by way of knowledge energy and vibration. Those who manipulate are also susceptible to manipulation for it is a sphere that has to be entered and therefore all is subject to the laws of manipulation. The master alchemist, exit the sphere of external relationships and enters a sphere of internal self The master manipulates the subtle elements within his/her self and their external environment and human relationships are transformed. This is the way of the master to which all who seek self-mastery (internal self) and work this way may acquire mastery. Guatema Buddha says. "The Masters' function is to help you remember who you are".

"Hotep ila antuk, Hotep ila kull Peace to you Peace to All"

Biography & Recommended Reading

Gerald Massey Egyptian Book of the Dead and the Mysteries of Amenta
The Sacred Records Of Neter: Aaferti Atum-Re" (Amunnubi Ruakh Ptah)
Hagukure The Book of the Samurai by Tsunemoto Yamamoto
Haru Hotep 'Solar Biology or Lunar Astrology'
Wayne B Chandler Ancient Future.
Ivan Van Sertima African Presence in Early Asia
N.K. Bose The Structure of Hindu Society
Ammonubi Roakhptah Dr Malachi Z York: Breaking The Spell,
Ammonubi Roakhptah Dr Malachi Z York: Our Bondage
Ammonubi Roakhptah Dr Malachi Z York: Your True Roots.
Ammonubi Roakhptah Dr Malachi Z York: Jesus Found In Egypt
The Handbook of Yoruba Religious concepts/Baba Ifa Karade
Amos Wilson: The falsification of African Consciousness.
Neely Fuller The United Independent compensatory code/system/concept a textbook/workbook for thought, speech and/or action for victims of racism (white supremacy)
Diodorus Siculus (*Author of Library of world history*)
For further reading about Black civilization and life in India between 10,000 BC to 1700BC "Susu Economics", published by http://www.authorhouse.com
"Wonderful Ethiopians of the Mighty Cushite Empire", by Drucilla Dunjee Houston, published by Black Classics Press, http://www.blackclassicspress.com (Baltimore, Maryland)
also http://www.cwo.com/~lucumi/runoko.html
Carlos Casteneda

Glossary and Definitions

A

Adresu	Learn
Afrika	A free Ka (spirit) Descendent of 9 ether/Solar beings and
Africa	to divide
African	Divided person
A'afrekan	African
Afrekeya	Africa
Agrub	Scorpion
Amun	Hidden One/Neter
Amenta	Duat, the abode of Neter and the soul/The unconscious
Ankh	Key to life/Key of the eternal
Anu	I Am/The Heavenly One
Anubu	Messenger of Heaven and Hell
Arush	Chakra
Arushaat	Chakras
Arat	Cobra
Asaru	"He who is seen" The Eye
Aset	Throne, Seat also known as Isis
Atum	The undifferentiated one/First borne of the deities
Atun	The unique one
Aum	(Nuwaubic) Sound of Life

B

Ba	"Strength, powerful" Soul
Bast	Cat/Fire
Bayna	Mid Breathing
Bes	Repeller of wrong doers

D

Djed	Stability
Djuhity	Tehuti/Thoth
Dub	Scarab beetle

E

Ennead	The Sacred Nine Neteru
Ethiopian	9 ether being, Kushite

Ether   Upper air, the medium of light and electromagnetism.

F
Farasha   Butterfly
Fug   High breathing

G
Ghaanum   Chanting

H
Hafuzyan   Guardian
Hanu   Movement
Hatha   Sun and Moon
Hekau   Words of power
Heru   "Far away"
Hery Heb   Egyptian Teachers
Het-Heru   The Dwelling house of Horus
Hudu   Afrikan Tai Chi
Hika   One of the constant companions of Re. Personification of miracles magic and the manipulation of elements and chemicals.
Huhi   The eternal breath
Hu   The force of creative will
Huwa   The creative force of will
Hotep   Peaceful, tranquil, satisfied

I
Isis   "Emotions"
Istamzaab   Position
Ifa   Yoruba Oracle system The cosmic intelligence of Yoruba cultural expression
Indus Kush   Name of Ancient name of India
In-perience   observation of internal feelings, internal actions and travels

K
Ka   "Double" Spirit
Kasub   Experience

Khat	Body
Khaybet	Plasmatic you
Kemet	The black one
Khemet	Land of the Blacks
Khemetic	Black culture
Khonsu	Traveler/Healer
Karast	Christ/anoint
Khu	"flail" mental
Kubru	Bridge
Kush	"Black" son of Ham the father of Nimrod. The name for Ethiopia before it was Abyssinia

M

Ma'at	Justice, order, rightousness/Female personification of wisdom
Manjet	The morning boat of Ra/Re
Meseket	The evening boat of Ra/Re
Mutalub	Student

N

Nefertem	Lotus 'beautiful completion' Young Temu
NTR	Neter Male/Female
Neter	Male personification of a deity
Netert	Female personification of a deity
Neteru	Guardians/Nature
Neb	Master
Nebu	Master
Nuwaubu	Right Knowledge, Right Wisdom, Right Overstanding, Sound Right Reasoning. "News bringer"
Nuwaubian	A person who prescribes to Right Knowledge, Right Wisdom, Right Overstanding, sound right reasoning. "A bringer of news"
Nubia	Land of the Nubians/Sudan
Nubun	Before the light, presenter of the news
Nun	The deep abyss
Nut	"Nurturer" Sky Netert

O

Osiris	"Lord of the perfect Black"
Orisha	(Yoruba) Neterian emanations of the creator manifesting through nature

Overstand	Oppose to understand to stand above a situation to get the 360 degrees of information and transcend.

P
Pa	The Definitive
Ptah	Opener 'one who opens the way'

R
Ragul	Exercise
Ragulaat	Exercises
Re	Sun/Father Sun deity
Ruwty	"Double headed lion" sphinx

S
Sakis	Bow & Arrow
Sanuy	Form/posture
Sanuyaat	Forms/postures
Sebek	
Sekhmet	The powerful, the mighty
Sem	Title of a priest 'Listener A Hearer'
Senta	Sister
Sena	Brother
Shen	To Encircle, infinity
Shu	"To Raise" light space dryness
Sia	Insight, incarnation of intuitive consciousness
Smai	Union

T
Tawi	Two lands
Tamare	Tamerri/name of Ancient Egypt/Afrika 'land of the sun'
Tamarean	Ancient Afrikan
Tamareyaat	Ancient Egyptians
Tao	The way, balance
Tarug	Path/Journey
Taruh	Hand
Tat	Low breathing
Taful	Prayer
Tehuti	Male personification of Wisdom/
Twa	People of Anu/the Twa Ptahrites/Pygmies

W

Waab   Spiritual priest

Y

Yaa   'Oh' summons, call upon

Printed in the United Kingdom
by Lightning Source UK Ltd.
127583UK00001B/45-62/P